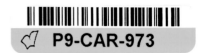

The GlucoseGoddess METHOD

JESSIE INCHAUSPÉ

SIMON
ELEMENT

TESTIMONIALS *from those who have tried* THE GLUCOSE GODDESS METHOD

"Having no more cravings is a huge game changer. I don't think about food all day long. I feel like a ball and chain have been cut off."

"Anyone who has a hard time sticking with a program should do this. The easy and gentle way into the hacks makes this so doable. Most diets are so strict that when one makes a mistake (which is 100% inevitable), one feels terrible and either binges to ease the disappointment or quits. As the hacks become a regular part of our day, we can slowly tailor the way we eat to accomplish what we need without feeling we are denying ourselves."

"I feel incredible. And to my surprise, I lost some weight around my belly—eating more than ever and even having dessert."

"My period is back after several years without it."

"I can't thank you enough. This program has changed my life completely!!"

"I feel so much better in all aspects. It's like I've become a different person and I couldn't be happier! I lost weight, my depression has decreased so much. It feels amazing, plus the brain fog is completely gone."

"I hadn't ovulated in over 5 months due to polycystic ovarian syndrome, and by following the Method I was able to ovulate and then get pregnant. I was about to start ovulation medication (Clomid), but thanks to doing this, it happened naturally. My husband and I are OVER THE MOON."

"I used to plan finishing my daily chores and errands by 2pm because I would crash afterwards. I could hardly move and often took a nap. Now I have energy all day long! It's incredible and I can't believe how much I can get done now."

"I had type 2 diabetes. I had previously been told by my dietician that, because I have coeliacs as well as diabetes, adjusting my metabolism would be like adjusting the course of an oil tanker. But I noticed results with this Method within 4 days. I continued beyond the 4 weeks, and my HbA1C dropped in 4 months from 9.6 to 4.7. I'm no longer diabetic at all. And I lost 25kg. This should be available through the government for anyone with prediabetes or diabetes."

"Surprisingly, one of the biggest differences I've noticed is in my skin! My acne has decreased dramatically. Kind of an unexpected but nice side effect :)"

"I have eczema and histamine intolerance. Both cause red rashes on my face and body. I could see a large improvement in them even in the first week."

"The best thing about this Method has been realising, at 55, that I can make changes to my diet that make me feel better, but don't feel punitive."

"Blood pressure lowered, hair loss reduced, lost weight, especially in the abdomen area. I am so grateful for these life-changing hacks! I know so many people who would benefit from this."

"My endocrinologist asked me what I did to improve my health, he couldn't believe how much better I am!"

"Anyone who feels slightly off kilter but can't identify why would benefit from this."

"This Method should be called: change your life in 4 steps."

"I have lost 2.8 kg in 4 weeks, the incredible thing is that it is waist and stomach fat. I had 6 kilos I wanted to lose for my health and now I'm halfway there. It's been nice and easy. I will continue to assimilate all these changes until I make them completely mine. Thank you."

"Every single person on earth would benefit from doing this Method."

"My relationship with food has changed completely. I LOVE that the Method does not demonise any type of food or craving, nothing needs to be cut out."

"My body feels great. Joints don't hurt so much. Cravings way down!"

"Going through perimenopause and I feel that these hacks have lessened the symptoms of feeling tired, low energy, brain fog, feeling hungry all the time."

"Thank you so much for this Method. I have felt so stuck for so long and now something has finally clicked and I am seeing results!"

CONTENTS

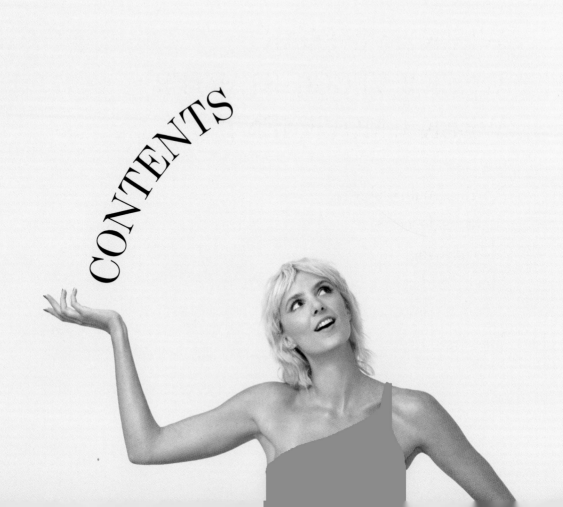

THE QUESTION THAT STARTED EVERYTHING

"Jessie, can you move in with me please?" The first time I was asked this question was in an Instagram message in May 2022—a few days after my first book, *Glucose Revolution*, came out. In that book, I shared the science of how blood sugar (also known as *glucose*) affects all aspects of our lives, and provided ten easy hacks to manage it in order to heal our bodies and get our happiness, energy, and health back.

So why did everybody suddenly want me as a roommate? Because many of you wanted more than my first book provided. You had taken onboard my research showing that the majority of us experience glucose spikes—rapid increases in blood sugar after eating—and that most of us didn't know it. You recognized the signs of glucose spikes in yourself (cravings, chronic fatigue, sugar addiction, poor sleep, inflammation, brain fog, polycystic ovary syndrome, diabetes, and many more). And you understood the hacks and loved how easy they were, but you wanted a plan to get started.

You wanted me by your side to help you put the science into practice, day by day, meal by meal. You wanted a workbook, recipes, encouragement, and inspiration. You wanted to know how other people had healed. You wanted help turning the glucose hacks into lifelong habits.

I jumped at this fantastic idea, sat down and got to work.

I thought about how I applied the hacks to my life when my glucose journey began four years ago. I thought about how I decided on the first hack. And then the second . . . I thought about how I chose what to buy at the grocery store, and about the first new dishes I cooked. I thought about what I say these days to friends who ask me for a step-by-step plan to start their glucose journey. I thought about what recipe I suggest to a family member who calls me for some inspiration. I thought about how I spoke to myself and what had motivated me along the way. I reached out to the readers of my first book and asked those who had successfully turned the hacks into habits what had helped them. Then I asked those who had found the hacks harder to sustain what they needed.

Out of this research came two things: First, lots of excitement on my part. Second, the book you are holding in your hands. I present to you . . . (drumroll please): *The Glucose Goddess Method*.

This actionable companion to *Glucose Revolution* consists of a four-week guide to help you incorporate the most important glucose hacks into your everyday life. It includes a step-by-step workbook that you can write in, a hundred of my favorite easy and delicious recipes, and answers to all your questions.

It is the equivalent of me moving in with you for four weeks, and showing you how to steady your glucose and feel better than ever. Learning how to reduce glucose spikes changed my life. And together, we are going to help you to thrive from the inside out so that you can show up as your optimal self and live your best life.

Congratulations for doing this and thank you for having me. I promise I'm a pretty good roommate.

THE 2,700-PERSON PILOT EXPERIMENT

From the very beginning of the Glucose Goddess movement in 2019, the involvement of the community has been phenomenal. For this book, I wanted to run a pilot experiment in which people would go through the Method, ask questions, and share their results. As I was putting together the recruitment form, I thought that a hundred people joining would be great... but to my surprise and delight, *thousands of you* volunteered.

Two thousand seven hundred amazing people have tried and tested the Glucose Goddess Method and helped make it the best it can possibly be. First, I'd like to thank them. You can find their names on pages 272–77, and lots of their quotes and tips throughout. They were from 110 countries, aged from 20 to 70 years old.

After the 4-Week Glucose Goddess Method:

90%
of participants
are less hungry

89%
of participants
have reduced
their cravings

77%
of participants
have more
energy

67%
of participants
are happier

58%
of participants
who wanted to
sleep better are
sleeping better

58%
of participants who
were struggling with
their mental health
have improved it

46%
of participants
who had skin
issues have seen
improvements
in their skin

41%
of participants who
wanted to improve
their diabetes have
improved it

35%
of participants
who were looking
to improve their
hormonal health
have improved it

During the course of this pilot experiment, dozens of women who weren't having their period anymore (a common symptom of glucose spikes) got their periods back, and three women who had been struggling to conceive for months got pregnant! I received countless messages telling of relationships improving, diabetes numbers getting better, lives changing. You can find more details about the study at glucosegoddess.com/method-whitepaper.

A note on weight loss

The Glucose Goddess Method is not a diet. Its objective is not weight loss. It is not restrictive, it does not ask you to count calories, and it actually asks you to eat more than usual. It is about health and healing your body from the inside out, and feeling amazing at any body size. But to many people's surprise, they actually lose weight while doing it, even while eating more than usual and not counting calories. That's because when we flatten our glucose curves, cravings dissipate, hormones rebalance, and we are in fat-burning mode more frequently and for longer. Weight loss is a common side effect of steadying our glucose levels. Of the 2,700 participants, **38 percent of people who wanted to lose weight did in fact lose weight in those four weeks.**

And, finally, 99 percent of people on the program said that they would be continuing with the hacks when the four-week study came to an end. They created new transformative habits for life. And so will you.

Before we dive right in, here are some of the basics of what you need to know.

Is the
GLUCOSE GODDESS
METHOD *for you?*

I used to believe that only people with diabetes needed to care about their glucose levels. In fact, everyone used to believe that. But reviewing the latest scientific progress showed me otherwise (you can find the references on page 278): the majority of the population experiences glucose spikes, which can lead to a wide range of symptoms and conditions. I like to think that these symptoms are our body speaking to us, trying to tell us about the glucose roller coaster happening within.

Ask yourself these questions to find out if you are experiencing glucose spikes, and if the Glucose Goddess Method can help you.

- Do you crave **sweet foods**?
- Are you "addicted to **sugar**"?
- Do you get **tired** throughout the day?
- Do you find it difficult to find the **energy** to do what you'd like to do?
- Do you need **caffeine** to keep you going through the day?
- Do you experience **brain fog**?
- Do you get a "**food coma**" after eating?
- Do you need to **eat every few hours**?
- Do you feel **agitated** or **angry** when you are hungry, aka *hangry*?
- Do you have **extreme hunger pangs** during the day?
- Do you feel **shaky, light-headed,** or **dizzy** if meals are delayed?
- Do you have **acne**?
- Do you have **eczema**?
- Do you have **psoriasis**?
- Do you suffer from **inflammation**?
- Do you have **endometriosis**?

- Do you have **polycystic ovary syndrome (PCOS)** or **missed periods**?
- Do you suffer from difficult **premenstrual syndrome** or **painful periods**?
- If you are female, are you experiencing **balding** on the head or **hair growth** on the face?
- Are you struggling with **fertility**?
- Are you trying to **lose weight** but finding it difficult?
- Do you have **trouble sleeping** or wake up with **heart palpitations**?
- Do you have **energy crashes** where you break out in a **sweat** or get **nauseous**?
- Do you experience **anxiety**?
- Do you experience **depression**?
- Do you experience any other **mental health** symptoms?
- Do you often find yourself becoming **irritated** by your friends and family for no obvious reason?
- Is your **mood variable**?
- Do you frequently get **colds**?
- Do you experience **acid reflux** or **gastritis**?
- Have you ever been told that your **glucose levels** are **elevated**?
- Do you have **reactive hypoglycemia**?
- Do you have **insulin resistance**?
- Do you have **prediabetes** or **type 2 diabetes**?
- Do you have difficulty managing **gestational diabetes**?
- Do you have difficulty managing **type 1 diabetes**?
- Do you have **nonalcoholic fatty liver disease**?
- Do you have **heart disease**?

And lastly (but perhaps most importantly) . . .

- Do you think you **could feel better** than you currently do?

If you answered yes to any of these questions, this Method is for you. Welcome!

What's GLUCOSE AGAIN?

Glucose is our body's preferred source of energy. Every cell in our body uses glucose to perform its function: our lung cells to breathe, our brain cells to think, our heart cells to pump blood, our eye cells to see, and so on. Glucose is important. And the main way we provide our bodies with glucose is by eating it. Glucose is found mostly in foods we call "carbohydrates" (or "carbs"): starchy foods (bread, pasta, rice, potatoes) and sugary foods (fruit, sweets, desserts).

You may think that if we need glucose for energy, more glucose will give us more energy, so we should try to eat as many sugary and starchy foods as possible, right? Actually, that's not the case: a plant needs *some* water to live but if you give it too much water, it dies. In the same way, give a human too much glucose and bad things start happening.

When we deliver too much glucose too quickly to our body after a meal, we experience what is called a *glucose spike*. This is not something that only affects people with diabetes. **Most of us experience glucose spikes** (about 80 percent of the population, according to some US estimates), and unfortunately, these spikes carry with them consequences that can harm our physical and mental health.

When we have lots of glucose spikes throughout a day, our blood-sugar level looks like this:

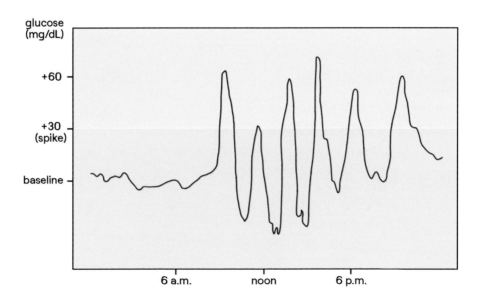

These spikes and drops leave us feeling tired, give us strong food cravings, and make us feel hungry every two hours; they are linked to inflammation, aging (and wrinkles!), low mood, hormonal imbalances that can result in difficult menopause symptoms, PCOS, brain fog … and in the long term, conditions such as type 2 diabetes and Alzheimer's. Scary, I know. But the good news is that we don't have to live with these symptoms.

How do we get off this roller coaster? We flatten the spikes. And this is where the hacks in this book come in.

When we incorporate the hacks, our glucose looks like this:

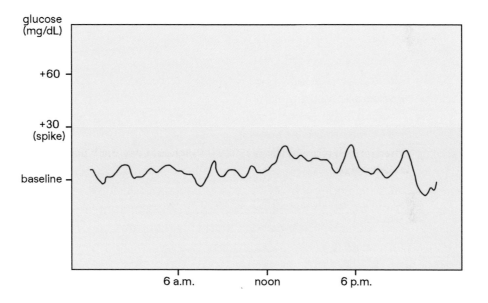

The beauty of it all is that the hacks that enable us to achieve these great results are easy. They do not ask you to go on a diet or cut out any foods. They are simple to implement, and once they are habits, you'll feel so good that you'll never want your day to go any other way.

FIRST, A BIT OF IMPORTANT SCIENCE . . .

Before we get to the hacks, I want you to be aware of what exactly happens in your body when you experience a glucose spike (and if you want to dive deeper, grab my first book, *Glucose Revolution*).

When we experience a glucose spike, it doesn't just happen in our bloodstream. Every single one of our cells, organs, and body parts feels it. Glucose disperses into every nook and cranny of our body, and three main processes are set in motion within us.

Mitochondria

First, our **mitochondria** (the powerhouses of our cells) **become overwhelmed**. These organelles are responsible for transforming glucose into energy for the body. But during a glucose spike, the amount of glucose coming their way becomes too much to handle. They become stressed and shut down. This leads to inflammation, and reduces their ability to make energy properly. Cue: chronic fatigue.

Glycation

Second, the more glucose spikes we experience, the faster we age. Glucose spikes accelerate a process called **glycation**, which is responsible for aging. It is actually similar to cooking, just like a chicken cooks in the oven. From the moment a human is born, they slowly cook (crazy, but true!) via this process of glycation. Then, when they are fully cooked, they die. Each glucose spike (especially those that come from sweet foods) accelerates glycation. This shows on our skin with wrinkles, and also internally as our organs slowly deteriorate. Glycation also increases inflammation, just like the first mitochondria-related process.

Insulin

Third, let's touch on insulin. Our body has a clever protection mechanism to shield us from some of the damage done by elevated glucose levels. During a glucose spike, **our pancreas sends out a hormone called insulin**, whose job it is to take glucose out of the bloodstream, to reduce the mitochondrial damage and glycation taking place. What does this insulin do with excess glucose? It stores it in our liver, muscles, and fat cells. This is one of the ways we gain fat on our body. And we should be thankful for this, because without insulin our body would be in a state of permanent crisis. The downside is that when insulin is present, fat-burning is deactivated. And over time, too much insulin carries with it its own consequences, such as the development of hormonal issues or type 2 diabetes.

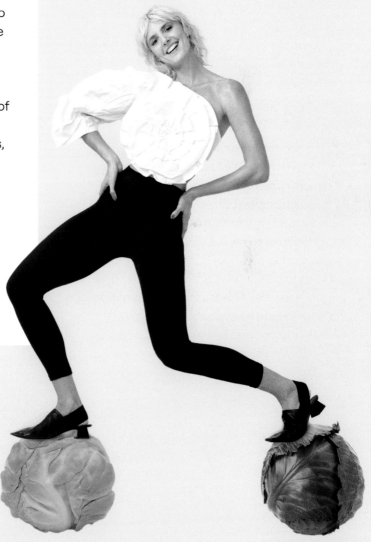

SYMPTOMS *and* CONDITIONS LINKED *to* GLUCOSE SPIKES

Glucose is so central to our body's functioning that an excess of it has repercussions for virtually every aspect of our physical and mental health. You may recognize a few of these in your own life.

Cravings

"I'm surprised how much my cravings have reduced. I always felt the need to eat huge amounts of chocolates, daily. Not anymore."

In 2011, a research team from Yale University changed our understanding of cravings. They placed people in an fMRI scanner, showed them photos of crave-worthy foods on a screen, and at the same time monitored their glucose levels. What the researchers discovered was fascinating. When the subjects' glucose levels were stable, everything looked normal. However, when their glucose levels were low, *the craving center of their brains lit up* and they rated the foods they were seeing much higher on the "I want to eat it" scale. This is what can happen during the crash after a glucose spike; we crave foods that we otherwise wouldn't care about. Steadying our curves, avoiding the spikes and the drops, keeps cravings at bay.

Chronic fatigue

"I've been suffering horribly with chronic fatigue, and for the first time in months, since starting this Method, I am finally starting to recover. These hacks are for life for me."

Let's go back to our mitochondria: the organelles responsible for making energy in our cells. Too much glucose makes them quit, which compromises energy production, and ultimately leaves us feeling tired. Studies show us that diets that cause glucose roller coasters lead to higher fatigue than those that flatten glucose curves. If you have damaged mitochondria, picking your kid up is more challenging, carrying groceries is exhausting, and you won't be able to handle stress as well as you used to. Mitochondria-generated energy is required to overcome difficult events, whether physical or mental.

Constant hunger

"I'm not hungry all the time, and I feel full faster. My food is more flavorful, too—is that a thing?"

Are you hungry all the time? You are not alone. And here again, it has to do with glucose. First, the short-term impact: if you compare two meals that contain the *same number of calories*, the one that leads to a smaller glucose spike will keep you feeling full for longer. So even if you don't change how many calories you eat, just focusing on your glucose levels will free you from constant hunger.

Second, the long-term impact: after years of glucose spikes, our hunger hormones get mixed up. Leptin, the hormone that tells us we are full and should stop eating, has its signal blocked; while ghrelin, the hormone that tells us we are hungry, takes over. Even though we have fat reserves, with lots of energy available, our body tells us we need more—so we eat. As we eat, we experience more glucose spikes, and insulin rushes in to store excess glucose as fat, which then increases the action of ghrelin. It's an unfortunate, vicious, and unfair cycle. The more weight we put on, the hungrier we get.

The answer is not to try to eat less; it is to decrease our insulin levels by flattening our glucose curves—and, spoiler alert, this often actually means eating *more* food, as you'll see in our Savory Breakfast and Veggie Starter weeks.

Weight gain

"I've lost 11 pounds so far, and I feel so much more energetic. I will continue this Method forever, it's become my new lifestyle."

Many of us have complicated feelings about fat, but it's actually very useful: our body uses its fat reserves to provide storage space for the excess glucose floating around in our bloodstream. This is one of the reasons that we gain weight. So, as I mentioned above, we shouldn't be mad at our body for putting on fat; instead, we should thank it for trying to protect us from glycation and inflammation.

That said, if you're trying to lose fat on your body, focusing on your glucose levels is a great way to do so. When you flatten your glucose curves, a few key things happen: First, cravings and hunger reduce. Second, because you have less insulin circulating in your body, you are in fat-burning mode more often.

While weight loss is not the primary objective of balancing our glucose levels, it is often a consequence.

Poor sleep

"It used to take me around one hour to fall asleep, but now I fall asleep in no time."

Sleep and glucose are very tightly linked: the more spikes we have, the worse our sleep is, and, if we are on a glucose roller coaster, we'll experience less restorative deep sleep. Going to bed with high glucose levels or right after a big glucose spike has also been shown to be associated with insomnia in postmenopausal women, and sleep apnea in a segment of the male population. Finally, a common symptom of dysregulated glucose is waking up suddenly in the middle of the night with a pounding heart. That can be the result of a glucose crash while we're asleep. And this is not all: after a bad night's sleep, you are more likely to have big glucose spikes after breakfast the next day. It's a vicious cycle. To put an end to it, start by flattening your curves.

Mental health

"I feel happier and my depression and anxiety seem more under control. I still have some ups and downs, but with better control."

Your brain doesn't have sensory nerves, so when something is wrong, it can't alert you with pain as other organs do. Instead, you feel mental disturbances—such as anxiety and poor mood. When people eat a diet that leads to erratic glucose levels, they report more depressive symptoms compared to those on a diet that leads to steadier glucose levels. And the symptoms get worse as the spikes get more extreme, so any effort to flatten the curve, even moderately, could help you feel better.

Mood

"I am so much less depressed and frustrated now. The difference is quite remarkable. And my relationship with my husband has improved."

Did you know that your glucose levels could influence your personality and your interactions with other people? In recent studies, scientists have been discovering fascinating connections: when our glucose levels are irregular, we are more likely to be irritated by our partner, and to punish those around us when they make a mistake. This is because glucose roller coasters can influence certain molecules in our brain affecting our mood: big spikes lead to lower tyrosine levels. Tyrosine is a neurotransmitter that is said to improve mood. And if you've ever experienced the feeling of being *hangry* (angry when hungry), there again, it is more common in people who have big glucose spikes and drops.

Brain fog

"Less brain fog has been my biggest improvement. This makes me super happy. The Method is now my new lifestyle. Not a diet."

Although glucose is an essential energy source for the brain, too much glucose harms it. First, several studies have shown that being on a glucose roller coaster for decades results in damage to our brain's blood vessels and our brain cells (neurons). This leads to decreased brain function and higher risk of stroke. Second, glucose roller coasters slow down the speed of signals between neurons. We often feel this as brain fog (difficulty concentrating, dizziness, confusion), memory issues, and poor cognitive function. Your brain will thank you for flattening your curves.

Gut health

"Since I started the Method, I haven't had digestion problems or bloating. And my stomach is flatter."

The gut is where our food is processed. It's no surprise, therefore, that bowel distress—such as leaky gut, irritable bowel syndrome, and slowed intestinal transit—is linked to diet. Remember how I said that glucose spikes increase inflammation throughout our organism? Well, inflammation is one of the things that can cause holes in the gut lining, which means that toxins that aren't supposed to get through do get through. This in turn can lead to leaky gut syndrome, gas, and bloating, but also drive food allergies and other autoimmune diseases, such as Crohn's disease and rheumatoid arthritis. Science is also showing us that when we eat in a way that causes many glucose spikes, the "bad" bacteria in our gut thrives, and the "good" bacteria decrease in number. This can cause a wide range of symptoms and general gut discomfort. If you're struggling with your gut health, it can be highly beneficial to flatten your glucose curves!

Wrinkles and aging

"I was worried about my future because I was aging faster than I should. I could feel it. All of the issues I was facing have either gone away or are lessening greatly. My doctors have been shocked."

Depending on your diet, you may have spiked your glucose thousands more times than your neighbor has by the time you reach 80. This will influence not only how old you look externally, but how old you are *internally*. Glycation and inflammation are responsible for the slow degradation of our cells: what we call aging.

These processes damage collagen, which causes sagging skin and wrinkles and can lead to inflammation in joints, rheumatoid arthritis, and the degradation of cartilage and osteoarthritis. The more often we spike, the faster we age.

Acne, rosacea, skin conditions

"I have eczema. It causes red rashes on my face and body. I could see a large improvement even in the first week of the Method. My skin heals much faster and my moisture barrier is much stronger."

Many skin conditions (including acne, rosacea, eczema, and psoriasis) are driven by inflammation, which, as you have learned, is a consequence of glucose spikes. When we eat in a way that flattens our glucose curves, inflammation is tamed, which helps acne clear up and pimples get smaller. In a study in males aged 15 to 25, the diet that resulted in the flattest glucose curves led to a significant reduction in acne. Getting glucose spikes under control can improve the health and appearance of our skin.

Fertility, PCOS, and hormonal issues

"My PMS, endometriosis, and adenomyosis symptoms reduced *amazingly* during the program. And after battling with PCOS to regulate my cycle since earlier this year . . . I got pregnant!!"

Whether it's polycystic ovary syndrome (PCOS), fibroids, endometriosis, menopause symptoms, PMS symptoms, missed periods . . . they all have to do with our hormonal system not working as it should. And the first thing to do to help our hormones function properly is to make sure our glucose levels are balanced. PCOS, in particular,

is becoming increasingly prevalent. In most cases, it is a disease caused by too much insulin. Why? Because insulin tells the ovaries to produce more testosterone (the male sex hormone). On top of that, with too much insulin, a natural conversion from male to female hormones that usually takes place is hampered—which leads to even more testosterone in the body. Because of the excess testosterone, females suffering from PCOS can display masculine traits: hair in places where they don't want hair (such as the chin), baldness, irregular or missed periods, or acne. Many women with PCOS also have a hard time losing weight—because where there is too much insulin, there is an inability to burn fat. The good news? In many cases, when insulin levels come back down, testosterone reduces, and PCOS symptoms go away.

Menopause

"My premenopause symptoms (sleep issues, lack of focus, hot flashes) have gone. I also lost five pounds that I was wanting to lose for so long—zero extra effort apart from these hacks."

The changes caused by the dramatic drop in hormone levels in menopause can feel like an earthquake—everything is thrown off-balance, and this process brings symptoms from reduced libido to night sweats, insomnia, hot flashes, and more. High or unstable glucose levels and high insulin levels make menopause feel worse. Research shows that hot flashes and night sweats are more likely in women who have high glucose and high insulin levels. But there's hope: a 2020 study from Columbia University found that flattening glucose curves is associated with fewer menopause symptoms.

Gestational diabetes

"I was diagnosed with gestational diabetes at 29 weeks pregnant. So far, huge changes: I feel better than I ever did. I'm not swollen, my glucose is steady, my doctor is happy, and, most importantly, I'm not scared anymore."

During every pregnancy, insulin levels increase in the body. That's because insulin is responsible for encouraging growth—growth of the baby and growth of the mother's breast tissue so she can prepare to breastfeed. But sometimes this extra insulin can lead to what's called *gestational diabetes*. By flattening their glucose curves, expectant mothers can reduce their likelihood of needing medication, prevent their baby from gaining excess weight in utero (which is good because it makes birth easier and is healthier for the baby), as well as limit their own weight gain during pregnancy and cut their risk of needing a C-section.

If you are expecting a baby, always check with your doctor that this Method is safe for you. (And during Week 2—vinegar week—make sure to look for pasteurized vinegar: most vinegars are pasteurized, but apple cider vinegar usually isn't.)

Sometimes, gestational diabetes actually points to the mother having had elevated glucose levels before pregnancy that weren't detected until the gestational diabetes test. This is why some mothers find their glucose levels are still elevated after they give birth; for these women, it's even more important to turn the glucose hacks into habits to solve the underlying issue.

Type 1 diabetes

"I have type 1 diabetes and my numbers have just been great! Thank you!"

Type 1 diabetes is an autoimmune condition in which affected people don't have the ability to make insulin—the cells in their pancreas that control its production don't work. Every time a person with type 1 diabetes experiences a glucose spike, their body cannot stash excess glucose in the usual storage units because there's no insulin to help. As a result, they need to inject themselves with insulin many times a day to compensate. But large spikes and dips are a daily, and stressful, challenge. By flattening their glucose curves, people with type 1 diabetes can lessen that challenge. If you have type 1 diabetes, it's important to speak to your doctor before you embark on this Method and to make sure your insulin dosage is adjusted if needed.

Insulin resistance, prediabetes, and type 2 diabetes

"In these four weeks my HbA1C has gone from 6.3 (prediabetic) to 5.7 (almost normal). I finally feel in control."

Type 2 diabetes is the most common form of diabetes, the root cause of which is insulin resistance (too much insulin circulating in the body for too long). Slowly but surely, over many years, every glucose spike we experience will contribute to increasing our insulin resistance and raising the overall baseline glucose level in our body. And, if that baseline gets too high, it leads to a diagnosis first of prediabetes and then type 2 diabetes.

It makes sense, therefore, that a diet that reduces your intake of glucose and consequently your production of insulin will help put type 2 diabetes into reverse. A 2021 review of 23 clinical trials made it clear that the most effective way to reverse type 2 diabetes is to flatten your glucose curves. This is more effective than low-calorie or low-fat diets, for example (even though they can also work). In 2019, the American Diabetes Association started endorsing glucose-flattening diets in light of mounting compelling evidence that these improve type 2 diabetes' outcomes. If you're looking to improve your type 2 diabetes, this Method will help you reduce your insulin levels, without giving up any of the foods you love. Let your doctor know before starting.

Cancer

"I feel empowered in my battle with breast cancer. I feel like I'm helping with this new way of eating."

Poor diet, together with smoking, is the main driver in 50 percent of cancers. For starters, research shows that cancer may begin with DNA mutations triggered by free radicals, which are, in turn, produced by stressed mitochondria and glycation. Second, inflammation promotes cancer's proliferation. Finally, when there is more insulin present, cancer spreads faster. By reducing glucose spikes, we slow down these three processes. The link between cancer and excess insulin shows in the data: people without diabetes have half the likelihood of dying from cancer compared to people with prediabetes. Always check with your care team if you are in the process of fighting cancer and want to use these hacks.

Alzheimer's and dementia

"Feeling more clear-headed, less brain fog. I've been able to focus on tasks better."

Of all the organs, the brain uses the most energy. It's home to a lot of mitochondria. This means that when there is excess glucose in our body, our brain is vulnerable to the consequences. The neurons in our brain feel the inflammation, glycation, and insulin resistance caused by too many glucose spikes. And, over time, the blood vessels in our brain also get damaged.

Alzheimer's and glucose levels are so closely connected that Alzheimer's is sometimes called "type 3 diabetes" or "diabetes of the brain." For example, people with type 2 diabetes are four times as likely to develop Alzheimer's as people without diabetes. And the signs are visible early: poorly controlled glucose in people with type 2 diabetes is associated with deficits in memory and learning. And new research shows that insulin resistance in mid-life (as early as 35 years old) is a predictor of cognitive decline in the future. Thus, keeping our baseline glucose low in early adulthood may reduce our risk of developing Alzheimer's disease.

As for the other symptoms and conditions mentioned here, it's possible that even cognitive decline is reversible: a growing number of studies show short-term and long-term improvements in memory and cognition when patients are put on a glucose-steadying diet.

THE FOUR HACKS
in this METHOD

In *Glucose Revolution*, my first book, I shared a total of *ten* science-backed hacks that help us curb glucose spikes (see box **below**). For this four-week plan, I place the spotlight on the four hacks that are the most important to start with. Why are they the most important to start with? Because they are the ones that will impact most powerfully on your glucose levels and your health. I will tell you about the others in the chapters to come, but these four are the fundamentals. They will instantly impact your glucose for the better—and all without asking you to change your food habits drastically, nor to count calories, nor to cut out anything from your life. They are the gentle giants that we all need in our back pockets, forever, getting us to a thriving place with relatively little effort.

The 10 Glucose Goddess Hacks, as presented in my first book, *Glucose Revolution*

I have highlighted in bold those we are focusing on in this Method.

- Eat foods in the right order (fiber, then proteins and fats, then starches and sugars)
- **Add a veggie starter to one meal a day**
- Stop counting calories
- **Have a savory breakfast**
- Eat any type of sugar you like—they're all the same
- Pick dessert over a sweet snack
- **Have one tablespoon of vinegar a day before the meal that will be highest in glucose**
- **After you eat, move**
- If you have to snack, go savory
- Put some "clothes" on your carbs (avoid eating starchy and sweet foods on their own—"clothe" them with protein, fat, or fiber to slow down glucose absorption; for example, have Greek yogurt with your brownie, or ham with your bread)

THE FOUR-WEEK PROGRAM

In Week 1, you will start having savory breakfasts. In Week 2, you will continue with your new breakfast and also welcome vinegar into your life. In Week 3, you will continue the first two hacks, and layer in veggie starters. Finally, Week 4 will see the addition of our fourth hack: moving after eating.

I have sequenced the hacks in this fashion for a reason—this is the most powerful progression for your glucose spikes to flatten and for you to feel the effects quickly.

I'll introduce these hacks one by one each week. And I will provide dozens of recipes to give you inspiration and help you to incorporate the hacks into your life. *But apart from adding these hacks, you can eat and do whatever you want.* I repeat: outside of these hacks, you can eat and do whatever you want. You can have all your usual favorite foods, eat sugar, drink alcohol.

At the end of the four weeks, it's up to you to decide whether you continue doing the hacks. My bet is that you will have found them so easy and powerful that they will become staples in your life. Let's meet them properly, shall we?

WEEK 1	DAY 1	DAY 2	DAY 3	DAY 4	DAY 5	DAY 6	DAY 7
	SAVORY BREAKFAST						

WEEK 2	DAY 8	DAY 9	DAY 10	DAY 11	DAY 12	DAY 13	DAY 14
	SAVORY BREAKFAST						
	VINEGAR once a day						

WEEK 3	DAY 15	DAY 16	DAY 17	DAY 18	DAY 19	DAY 20	DAY 21
	SAVORY BREAKFAST						
	VINEGAR once a day						
	VEGGIE STARTER once a day						

WEEK 4	DAY 22	DAY 23	DAY 24	DAY 25	DAY 26	DAY 27	DAY 28
	SAVORY BREAKFAST						
	VINEGAR once a day						
	VEGGIE STARTER once a day						
	10-MINUTE MOVEMENT after a meal						

WEEK 1: SAVORY BREAKFAST

It's a common assumption that eating something sweet for breakfast will give us energy. But that's actually not true. While sugar at breakfast gives us *pleasure*, it is not the best way to give us *energy*. A glucose spike from a sweet breakfast harms our mitochondria (cue: fatigue), and because of the action of insulin rushing in to stash glucose away, at equal calories, a sweet breakfast actually gives our body *less* energy than a savory one.

Unfortunately, a typical Western diet leans toward breakfasting on glucose-spiking foods such as cereal, toast and jam, croissants, granola, pastries, sweet oats, biscuits, fruit juice, Pop-Tarts, fruit smoothies, acai bowls, and so on. All of these foods are composed of mostly starch and sugar: big, big glucose spikes, and with them, consequences for the rest of our day.

Week 1 of the Glucose Goddess Method will say goodbye to glucose spikes for breakfast, and in so doing will offer you a completely new experience of your days: no cravings and steady energy.

How do we do it? In Week 1, **we have a savory breakfast every day.**

Answers to all your questions, tips and advice from the community, recipes, and advice on how to make your own savory breakfast start on page 36.

WEEK 2: VINEGAR

During Week 2, you will continue with the savory breakfast hack, and add in another. This one won't require you to change anything that you are eating, you will simply be welcoming into your daily habits one tablespoon of our dear friend vinegar.

Vinegar has been used for generations as a health ingredient—notably in countries like Iran, where making it at home and having some every day is the norm. In the eighteenth century it was even prescribed as a tea for people with diabetes.

Since then, scientists have worked out exactly why vinegar is so good for us. And let me tell you, it's very cool.

Studies have shown that one tablespoon of vinegar can reduce the glucose spike of a meal by up to 30 percent. And the insulin spike by up to 20 percent. With that, cravings are curbed, hunger is tamed, and more fat is burned. This is a very cheap trick, too: a standard bottle of vinegar costs less than $5 and contains more than 60 one-tablespoon servings. You're welcome.

Starting in Week 2, **your goal will be to have one tablespoon of vinegar per day**. You will find many recipe ideas in this book to inspire you, from the most simple, the GG Classic—vinegar in water (with a straw, to protect your teeth)—to my favorite warming teas and party mocktails.

There are more details and answers to questions, like whether you can drink vinegar while pregnant and so on, starting on page 94.

WEEK 3: VEGGIE STARTER

In Week 3, we will continue with our savory breakfast and vinegar, and now add in the fabulous *Veggie Starter*. This means **adding a vegetable-based dish to the beginning of lunch or dinner**.

Why? Because vegetables contain a powerful component called *fiber*. When eaten at the beginning of a meal, fiber significantly reduces the glucose spike of any food that follows. The mechanism by which it performs this feat is amazing: as fiber arrives in our intestines, it deploys itself against our intestinal walls. There, it forms a protective mesh that slows and *reduces* the absorption into the bloodstream of any glucose coming down afterward.

You can eat anything you usually eat after your veggie starter, knowing that because the fiber mesh is there, there will be less of a glucose spike from your meal.

Veggie starters can be as simple as raw veggies from the fridge (page 150), or as fancy as slow-cooked leeks (page 186). Ideally, **try to make the veggie starter comprise about 30 percent of your meal**. I have more than 30 veggie starter recipes for you in Week 3, all more simple and delicious than the one before. *And* I have prepared veggie starter recipes that **also include vinegar**: if you choose them, or if you add your own vinegar dressing to your veggie starter, you'll check off two hacks in one.

You can find answers to all your questions starting on page 140.

WEEK 4: MOVING AFTER EATING

Last, but certainly not least . . . is Week 4, in which we recruit our most powerful allies on our journey to steady glucose: our muscles! It's time to wake them up to their newfound role.

The more and the harder a muscle contracts, the more energy it needs. The more energy it needs, the more glucose it needs.

The rate of glucose burning varies widely depending on how hard we're working—that is, how much energy our muscles require. It can increase a thousandfold from when we are at rest (sitting on our couch watching TV) to when we are intensely exercising (sprinting to catch our dog running across the park). But with every new muscle contraction, we burn up glucose molecules. And we can use this simple equation to our advantage to flatten our glucose curves.

Week 4 will ask you to continue with your daily savory breakfast, vinegar, and veggie starter, and to also **use your muscles for 10 minutes after one meal each day**, within 90 minutes after the end of that meal.

Answers to all your questions start on page 216.

YOU *may be* WONDERING . . .

Can I join a group doing the Method?

You sure can, and it will probably be really beneficial. During the 2,700-person pilot experiment, I received feedback that people *loved* doing the Method in a group, where they were held accountable and could share their difficulties and encourage each other. So I put something together online: you can join other people doing the Glucose Goddess Method on my website at glucosegoddess.com/method-group, or by scanning the QR code below. It's a fun experience that will leave you motivated and feeling connected to others around the world. You'll get support, encouragement, and community. The experience comes complete with videos of me walking you through the different steps of the four-week plan.

Do I need to wear a continuous glucose monitor?

No, you don't. I use data from my continuous glucose monitor to illustrate scientific concepts (the graphs you will find in this book and those on my Instagram, @glucosegoddess, all come from it). You don't need to wear one yourself. However, if you do have one, that's totally fine, and it may be interesting for you to watch in real time as your glucose levels steady during the Method.

Do I have to follow your recipes?

No. The recipes are just ideas, there to help and inspire you—and I'd be so happy to know that you've taken them as inspiration and created your own. I provide principles at the beginning of each week to guide you.

Do you have vegetarian, vegan, gluten-free options?

Yes! I've noted which recipes are vegetarian, vegan, and/or gluten-free at the end of each recipe.

Can I eat out?

Yes. At the beginning of each week, I give you some pointers on how to do the hacks if you are not eating at home.

What if there is a day when I can't follow the Method? Do I have to do the hacks every day?

Ideally, yes. The more you do the hacks, the more you'll see results. But the Method will still work if you do the hacks 80 percent of the time. Missing the odd day is no big deal. These are lifelong habits you are creating, and some days they will be difficult to see through.

Are there off-limits foods?

No foods are off-limits. Just follow the hacks; the rest of the time you can eat absolutely what you want, and, yes, that also means dessert and pizza. Breakfast is the only meal where there will be no sweet foods, except whole fruit to taste, but you can eat that anytime during the rest of the day.

Can I still drink alcohol?

Yes, you can eat and drink whatever you normally eat and drink. Because I am often asked this question, here are more details on alcohol: Spirits mixed with soda water, and wine (any color) are the best options to keep your glucose steady. Cocktails and beer are less favorable and more likely to cause a spike. That said, my philosophy is that if you're going to drink alcohol, it's not a health decision (there are no health benefits to alcohol), it's a *pleasure* decision. So pick the alcohol that you prefer.

I'm allergic to something in the recipes; is it okay to remove it or replace it?

Yes, absolutely.

Can I add or modify the recipes?

Yes, just don't add any sugar to them.

Should I stop my medication?

No—never without speaking to your doctor. And in fact, if you are on any kind of medication, you should tell your doctor about this Method and show them what you're going to be doing before you begin.

What if I already do the hacks?

Awesome! No worries. You can keep doing them or start from scratch again, starting with the savory breakfast in Week 1, adding in vinegar in Week 2, and so on. It's up to you.

Do I need to count calories or cut out things?

No! You just have to add the hacks into your life. The rest of the time, live your life freely.

Can I add more hacks more quickly?

Sure! But you don't need to.

What day of the week should I start?

Any day. How about tomorrow?

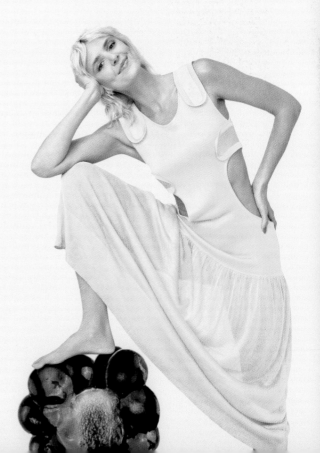

NOTES ABOUT THE RECIPES
and Bonus Content

The first three weeks are complete with tons of fun, easy recipes. Feel free to pick any of them to complete the hacks for that day. I've kept things super simple—not too many ingredients, not too time-consuming. And very delicious. Here is some extra information to help you.

What I expect you to have in your pantry
Salt, pepper, olive oil, access to tap water

Grocery shopping
I have not made grocery shopping lists for each week, because there is a lot of freedom in how you can go about choosing recipes. **The best way to set yourself up for success is to plan ahead and to make your own grocery list.** For Week 1 you need ingredients for savory breakfasts. So have a look at which ones you want to try, or think of your own savory breakfast ideas, and buy the ingredients for those.

Because I know some of you will find this helpful, I went ahead and created an example grocery shopping list, selecting some of my current favorite recipes. You can access it at glucosegoddess.com/method-grocery or by scanning the QR code below.

Gluten-free, vegetarian, and vegan recipes
You will see *gluten-free, vegetarian*, and *vegan* marked at the end of each recipe. This is not because one is better than the others, it is simply to make your life easier if you follow any of these specific diets. I've treated all cheeses as vegetarian, even though sometimes cheeses are made using animal enzymes and so are not strictly vegetarian. Again, I've gone for simplicity.

Avocados
Where a recipe calls for half an avocado, leave the pit in the unused half, and wrap it in foil. You can then refrigerate it for up to 24 hours.

Bonus content at the end of the book
At the end of this book, you'll find some bonus recipes to use whenever you want: **main dishes and desserts** (yes, we can have dessert!). I've created them so that they will keep your glucose levels steady. The anytime main dishes and desserts have one key thing in common: you'll never find sugar and starches in them on their own—I always put "clothes" on them. That means that whenever a recipe contains sugars and starches, it will also contain fat, protein, or fiber (or all three), which are key to keeping us steady.

And finally, I have included a cheat sheet for what to do if a craving hits, and you'll also find a list of all the scientific papers that are the basis for this Method.

THE WORKBOOK
Starting on the next page

We're adding a new glucose hack to our lives every week for four weeks, which is a lot of new things. So you may find it helpful to have a place to keep track of everything (I definitely do). This is why I created this workbook (see overleaf).

It will assist you in keeping track of how you are feeling with each hack, so you can begin to connect the flattening of your glucose levels with changing symptoms and improvements. You can start the workbook on any day of the week. There is no difference between weekdays and weekends. When rating how you feel on the scale from 1 to 5, 5 represents the strongest. I recommend you briefly scan through it to see what's ahead of you.

When you've decided what day you will start the Method, write down the date where indicated. Then return to this workbook every day to track your progress. Feel free to write directly on these pages with a pen or if you'd like to download additional versions (maybe for someone you're doing this with), you can do so for free at glucosegoddess.com/method-workbook, or scan the QR code below:

WEEK 1: SAVORY BREAKFAST

DAY 1 | DATE:

SAVORY BREAKFAST

How did you feel today? 🙂 ☺ 😐 ☹ 😞

How strong were your cravings? ....
(ON A SCALE OF 1–5)

How much energy did you have? ....
(ON A SCALE OF 1–5)

Your space for notes: ....
....
....
....
....
....
....
....

DAY 2 | DATE:

SAVORY BREAKFAST

How did you feel today? 🙂 ☺ 😐 ☹ 😞

How strong were your cravings? ....
(ON A SCALE OF 1–5)

How much energy did you have? ....
(ON A SCALE OF 1–5)

Your space for notes: ....
....
....
....
....
....
....
....

DAY 3 | DATE:

SAVORY BREAKFAST

How did you feel today? 🙂 ☺ 😐 ☹ 😞

How strong were your cravings? ....
(ON A SCALE OF 1–5)

How much energy did you have? ....
(ON A SCALE OF 1–5)

Your space for notes: ....
....
....
....
....
....
....
....

DAY 4 | DATE:

SAVORY BREAKFAST

How did you feel today? 🙂 ☺ 😐 ☹ 😞

How strong were your cravings? ....
(ON A SCALE OF 1–5)

How much energy did you have? ....
(ON A SCALE OF 1–5)

Your space for notes: ....
....
....
....
....
....
....
....

WEEK 1: SAVORY BREAKFAST

DAY 5 | DATE:

SAVORY BREAKFAST

How did you feel today? 🙂 🙂 😐 🙁 ☹️

How strong were your cravings? ....
(ON A SCALE OF 1–5)

How much energy did you have? ....
(ON A SCALE OF 1–5)

Your space for notes: ....
....
....
....
....
....
....

DAY 6 | DATE:

SAVORY BREAKFAST

How did you feel today? 🙂 🙂 😐 🙁 ☹️

How strong were your cravings? ....
(ON A SCALE OF 1–5)

How much energy did you have? ....
(ON A SCALE OF 1–5)

Your space for notes: ....
....
....
....
....
....
....

DAY 7 | DATE:

SAVORY BREAKFAST

How did you feel today? 🙂 🙂 😐 🙁 ☹️

How strong were your cravings? ....
(ON A SCALE OF 1–5)

How much energy did you have? ....
(ON A SCALE OF 1–5)

Your space for notes: ....
....
....
....
....
....
....

SUMMARY

Which of these have improved since you started the Method?

Mood   Energy   Hunger
Cravings   Sleep   Skin

Other things you noticed in your physical and mental health?
....
....

What was the most difficult part of this week?
....
....

What was your favorite savory breakfast?
....
....

WEEK 2: VINEGAR

DAY 8 | DATE:

SAVORY BREAKFAST
VINEGAR once a day

How did you feel today? 🙂 🙂 😐 🙁 ☹️

How strong were your cravings? ....
(ON A SCALE OF 1–5)

How much energy did you have? ....
(ON A SCALE OF 1–5)

Your space for notes: ....
....
....
....
....
....

DAY 9 | DATE:

SAVORY BREAKFAST
VINEGAR once a day

How did you feel today? 🙂 🙂 😐 🙁 ☹️

How strong were your cravings? ....
(ON A SCALE OF 1–5)

How much energy did you have? ....
(ON A SCALE OF 1–5)

Your space for notes: ....
....
....
....
....
....

DAY 10 | DATE:

SAVORY BREAKFAST
VINEGAR once a day

How did you feel today? 🙂 🙂 😐 🙁 ☹️

How strong were your cravings? ....
(ON A SCALE OF 1–5)

How much energy did you have? ....
(ON A SCALE OF 1–5)

Your space for notes: ....
....
....
....
....
....

DAY 11 | DATE:

SAVORY BREAKFAST
VINEGAR once a day

How did you feel today? 🙂 🙂 😐 🙁 ☹️

How strong were your cravings? ....
(ON A SCALE OF 1–5)

How much energy did you have? ....
(ON A SCALE OF 1–5)

Your space for notes: ....
....
....
....
....
....

WEEK 2: VINEGAR

DAY 12 | DATE:

> **SAVORY BREAKFAST VINEGAR** once a day

How did you feel today? 😀 🙂 😐 🙁 ☹️

How strong were your cravings? ....
(ON A SCALE OF 1–5)

How much energy did you have? ....
(ON A SCALE OF 1–5)

Your space for notes: ....
....
....
....
....
....

DAY 13 | DATE:

> **SAVORY BREAKFAST VINEGAR** once a day

How did you feel today? 😀 🙂 😐 🙁 ☹️

How strong were your cravings? ....
(ON A SCALE OF 1–5)

How much energy did you have? ....
(ON A SCALE OF 1–5)

Your space for notes: ....
....
....
....
....
....

DAY 14 | DATE:

> **SAVORY BREAKFAST VINEGAR** once a day

How did you feel today?

How strong were your cravings? ....
(ON A SCALE OF 1–5)

How much energy did you have? ....
(ON A SCALE OF 1–5)

Your space for notes: ....
....
....
....
....
....

SUMMARY

Which of these have improved since you started the Method?

Mood   Energy   Hunger
Cravings   Sleep   Skin

Other things you noticed in your physical and mental health?
....
....

What was the most difficult part of this week?
....
....

What was your favorite way of having vinegar?
....
....

WEEK 3: VEGGIE STARTER

DAY | DATE:
15 |

SAVORY BREAKFAST
VINEGAR once a day
VEGGIE STARTER once a day

How did you feel today? 🙂 🙂 😐 🙁 ☹️

How strong were your cravings? ....
(ON A SCALE OF 1–5)

How much energy did you have? ....
(ON A SCALE OF 1–5)

Your space for notes: ....
....
....
....

DAY | DATE:
16 |

SAVORY BREAKFAST
VINEGAR once a day
VEGGIE STARTER once a day

How did you feel today? 🙂 🙂 😐 🙁 ☹️

How strong were your cravings? ....
(ON A SCALE OF 1–5)

How much energy did you have? ....
(ON A SCALE OF 1–5)

Your space for notes: ....
....
....
....

DAY | DATE:
17 |

SAVORY BREAKFAST
VINEGAR once a day
VEGGIE STARTER once a day

How did you feel today? 🙂 🙂 😐 🙁 ☹️

How strong were your cravings? ....
(ON A SCALE OF 1–5)

How much energy did you have? ....
(ON A SCALE OF 1–5)

Your space for notes: ....
....
....
....

DAY | DATE:
18 |

SAVORY BREAKFAST
VINEGAR once a day
VEGGIE STARTER once a day

How did you feel today? 🙂 🙂 😐 🙁 ☹️

How strong were your cravings? ....
(ON A SCALE OF 1–5)

How much energy did you have? ....
(ON A SCALE OF 1–5)

Your space for notes: ....
....
....
....

WEEK 3: VEGGIE STARTER

DAY 19 | DATE:

> SAVORY BREAKFAST
> VINEGAR once a day
> VEGGIE STARTER once a day

How did you feel today? ☺ ☺ ☺ ☹ ☹

How strong were your cravings? ....
(ON A SCALE OF 1–5)

How much energy did you have? ....
(ON A SCALE OF 1–5)

Your space for notes: ....
....
....
....

DAY 20 | DATE:

> SAVORY BREAKFAST
> VINEGAR once a day
> VEGGIE STARTER once a day

How did you feel today? ☺ ☺ ☺ ☹ ☹

How strong were your cravings? ....
(ON A SCALE OF 1–5)

How much energy did you have? ....
(ON A SCALE OF 1–5)

Your space for notes: ....
....
....
....

DAY 21 | DATE:

> SAVORY BREAKFAST
> VINEGAR once a day
> VEGGIE STARTER once a day

How did you feel today? ☺ ☺ ☺ ☹ ☹

How strong were your cravings? ....
(ON A SCALE OF 1–5)

How much energy did you have? ....
(ON A SCALE OF 1–5)

Your space for notes: ....
....
....
....

SUMMARY

Which of these have improved since you started the Method?

Mood   Energy   Hunger
Cravings   Sleep   Skin

Other things you noticed in your physical and mental health?
....
....

What was the most difficult part of this week?
....
....

What was your favorite veggie starter?
....
....

WEEK 4: MOVING AFTER EATING

DAY | DATE:
22

SAVORY BREAKFAST
VINEGAR once a day
VEGGIE STARTER once a day
MOVING after a meal

How did you feel today? 🙂 🙂 😐 🙁 ☹️

How strong were your cravings? ....
(ON A SCALE OF 1–5)

How much energy did you have? ....
(ON A SCALE OF 1–5)

Your space for notes: ....
....
....

DAY | DATE:
23

SAVORY BREAKFAST
VINEGAR once a day
VEGGIE STARTER once a day
MOVING after a meal

How did you feel today? 🙂 🙂 😐 🙁 ☹️

How strong were your cravings? ....
(ON A SCALE OF 1–5)

How much energy did you have? ....
(ON A SCALE OF 1–5)

Your space for notes: ....
....
....

DAY | DATE:
24

SAVORY BREAKFAST
VINEGAR once a day
VEGGIE STARTER once a day
MOVING after a meal

How did you feel today? 🙂 🙂 😐 🙁 ☹️

How strong were your cravings? ....
(ON A SCALE OF 1–5)

How much energy did you have? ....
(ON A SCALE OF 1–5)

Your space for notes: ....
....
....

DAY | DATE:
25

SAVORY BREAKFAST
VINEGAR once a day
VEGGIE STARTER once a day
MOVING after a meal

How did you feel today? 🙂 🙂 😐 🙁 ☹️

How strong were your cravings? ....
(ON A SCALE OF 1–5)

How much energy did you have? ....
(ON A SCALE OF 1–5)

Your space for notes: ....
....
....

WEEK 4: MOVING AFTER EATING

DAY | DATE:
26

SAVORY BREAKFAST
VINEGAR once a day
VEGGIE STARTER once a day
MOVING after a meal

How did you feel today? 😃 🙂 😐 🙁 😫

How strong were your cravings? ....
(ON A SCALE OF 1–5)

How much energy did you have? ....
(ON A SCALE OF 1–5)

Your space for notes: ....
....
....

DAY | DATE:
27

SAVORY BREAKFAST
VINEGAR once a day
VEGGIE STARTER once a day
MOVING after a meal

How did you feel today? 😃 🙂 😐 🙁 😫

How strong were your cravings? ....
(ON A SCALE OF 1–5)

How much energy did you have? ....
(ON A SCALE OF 1–5)

Your space for notes: ....
....
....

DAY | DATE:
28

SAVORY BREAKFAST
VINEGAR once a day
VEGGIE STARTER once a day
MOVING after a meal

How did you feel today? 😃 🙂 😐 🙁 😫

How strong were your cravings? ....
(ON A SCALE OF 1–5)

How much energy did you have? ....
(ON A SCALE OF 1–5)

Your space for notes: ....
....
....

SUMMARY

Which of these have improved since you started the Method?

Mood   Energy   Hunger
Cravings   Sleep   Skin

Other things you noticed in your physical and mental health?
....
....

What was the most difficult part of this week?
....
....

What was your favorite movement?
....
....

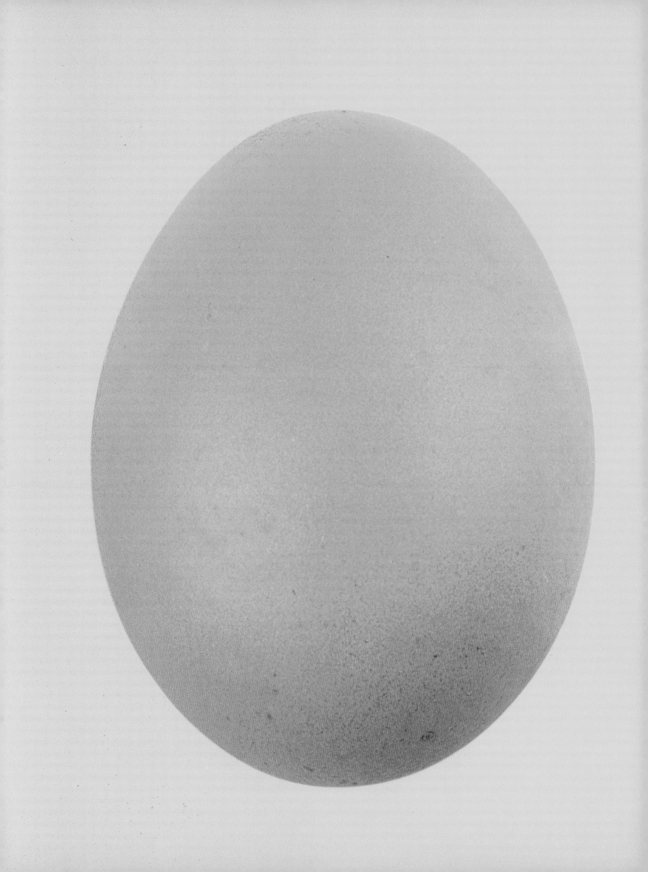

SAVORY BREAKFAST

And so we begin! First things first, we're going to unpack the most powerful meal of the day: breakfast.

TESTIMONIALS FROM THE COMMUNITY

"I don't know where to start! I feel unbelievably good! And after just one week! I can't wait for the rest of the program. I'm bursting with energy and laughing and dancing. I don't get hangry anymore."

"Changing my breakfast from sweet to savory has set my day on a whole new trajectory."

"I used to be always tired and I ate a lot of sweets, which made me feel guilty. Now it's hard for me to believe that such a simple change changed so much. First of all, I have energy all day long—I do not feel like sleeping at all—and, most importantly, the desire for sweets is very much fixed, even though I had a huge problem with it. I have will and energy back! And now, even though I get up to feed my youngest child in the middle of the night, I wake up full of energy instead of feeling dead like I did before!"

"I can concentrate very well on my work. I work for my father and he said yesterday (day six!) that he notices that I am doing well! That makes me really happy."

"I really notice an incredible difference in my energy level the last few days. Getting out of my bed was always really difficult, no matter how long I slept, and I dragged myself through the day. But now what a difference: I jump out of bed in the morning! And even after a full working day, I still have a lot of energy left. I also notice that I sleep more peacefully. (All this is without sleeping longer.)"

"The main thing that has improved is that I don't feel so hungry; I can wait. And also I'm less anxious. I can tell, without exploding, what bothers me."

"What helped me is seeing and feeling the results. Once you feel change, it jump-starts something in you and motivates you. It makes you trust what you're doing—you know it isn't a gimmick. With these hacks, you will see immediate results most of the time, even if they're small. For me, the first one was not falling asleep right after eating. The second one was not bloating. That did it for me."

"My behavior with my children is much more Zen after this week. I'm less stressed out."

"Would now not even consider anything but a savory breakfast to start my day. I love how nonjudgmental this Method is. I feel really encouraged."

"I used to think that I needed a lot of carbs in the morning to have energy and be satiated for longer . . . but I learned that I was wrong. I'm happy with the savory breakfasts, and I have the energy to work and be creative all day. I'm on fire!!!! I still have some cravings but I'm able to control them and not the other way around. . . . Life-changing."

"After this first week, I'm eating with much less guilt and my body sends me sensations of physical hunger again . . . this makes me almost cry with emotion after a lot of years of a bad relationship with food."

"I used to have cravings between meals. And couldn't resist most of the time. Now I eat breakfast and don't think of food until lunchtime."

"I used to always need a morning snack, but now I'm not hungry until at least 12 or 1 p.m. If given the opportunity to have something sweet at breakfast, I feel like I don't really need it and have loved sticking to savory, which is rare for me! I would often start with savory then add a pancake or piece of toast with jam and peanut butter at the end, and now I don't feel it's necessary."

"In just one week my skin and my hair look better. I feel peaceful and sleep better."

"My doctor informed me last month that I urgently needed to work on my stress levels or I would have to start taking medication. I couldn't get myself to do anything because I had no energy. After Week 1 of this Method, the only change has been the savory breakfast, and I feel like I'm on top of the world! It's having a big impact on my stress. I'm feeling so good."

"I often wear a smart watch that somehow measures my stress level. Until recently I had an average score of 60–70 (high stress score). Today, day 7, my stress score was 21! You can see a gigantic plunge in the graph! Plus everything is so tasty and quick to prepare."

Your objective for Week 1

Your objective during this first week is to eat a savory breakfast every day. Why? Because a savory breakfast is the cornerstone of a day of steady glucose, which will allow your whole day to go much more smoothly than before.

In this chapter, I will explain in detail what a savory breakfast is (a meal built around protein and fat, and one that includes nothing sweet except whole fruit) and share many of my favorite recipes. Ideally, you will find recipes that you like and can quickly make in the morning. You're going to continue having a savory breakfast every day for the whole length of the Method (the next four weeks), so my advice is to experiment until you fall in love with a few recipes that you can easily repeat.

Having made sure your breakfast is a savory one (and more on how to do that on page 42), you can eat whatever you want for the rest of the day. And if cravings come up, don't try to suppress or resist them. We aren't here to restrict any foods. Eat whatever you like. **You'll notice that as your glucose levels steady with this new hack, your cravings will naturally subside.** That's what happens when we fix the glucose roller coaster that was causing the cravings in the first place.

The science

As I touched on in the introduction, despite the long-held assumption that eating something sweet or starchy for breakfast (cereal, muesli, cereal bars, fruit juices, bread, fruit smoothies, oats, pastries) is important to give our body energy, in fact, the opposite is the case. Science shows us that, **while a sweet and starchy breakfast gives us *pleasure* (it releases dopamine in our brain), it is not the best way to give us *energy*.** A sweet and starchy breakfast leads to a glucose spike, which hurts our body's ability to make energy efficiently, makes us tired, and kicks off all kinds of side effects.

And that's not all: **a breakfast glucose spike will make us hungry again sooner**; and the bigger the breakfast spike, the bigger the drop after it, and therefore the worse the hunger and cravings will be. This kind of breakfast will also deregulate our glucose levels for the rest of the day, so our lunch and dinner, in turn, will create bigger spikes.

On top of all *that*, **first thing in the morning, when we are in our fasted state, our bodies are at their most sensitive to glucose**. Our stomach is empty, so anything that lands in it will be digested extremely quickly, which is why eating sugars and starches at breakfast often leads to the biggest spike of the day. Breakfast is the *worst time* to eat just sugar and starches, yet it's the time at which most of us do exactly that.

You may not yet have traced the symptoms you feel throughout the day back to your breakfast. And no wonder—because we don't instantly feel the effect that a spiky breakfast has on us. If, as soon as we ate that bowl of cereal, we were to have a panic attack and then fall asleep at the table, we'd get it. But because metabolic processes take hours to unfold, compound over time, and become mixed with all the other things that happen in a day, connecting the dots takes a bit of detective work—at least until we get the hang of it.

During this week, this is what you will discover: switching from a sweet and starchy to a savory breakfast will leave you feeling like a whole new person. Yes, seriously!

With a savory breakfast, symptoms you may have been feeling your whole life will start to dissipate. You'll unlock energy in your cells, prevent your brain from falling into craving cycles, and tame your hunger levels. You'll also create smaller spikes for lunch and dinner, creating a virtuous cycle.

Turn this hack into a habit and you will be well on your way to changing everything. So let's get to it.

The amazing steadiness that a savory breakfast (here, omelet and avocado) creates in our body

How to make a savory breakfast

All of the recipes on the following pages pass the test of a savory breakfast that will keep your glucose steady. I hope you'll find several that you love. Here's what all savory breakfasts have in common:

• **They are built around protein.** Protein is the centerpiece of a savory breakfast—it's what keeps you steady, full, and satiated. Your glucose levels *love* protein. Take your pick: Greek yogurt, tofu, meat, cold cuts, fish, cheese, cream cheese, protein powder, nuts, nut butter, seeds, and, yes, eggs (scrambled, fried, poached, or boiled).

• **They contain fat.** Scramble your eggs in butter or olive oil and add slices of avocado, or add five almonds, chia seeds, or flaxseeds to your Greek yogurt. Skip the fat-free yogurt and switch to 5% fat Greek yogurt. Fat is very important and not to be feared. (If you have questions about fat and heart health, head to my first book, *Glucose Revolution*, chapter 7.)

• **They contain fiber when possible.** It can be challenging to include fiber in the morning because it means eating veggies for breakfast. I don't blame you if you aren't into that. But if you can, do it. I love mixing spinach into my scrambled eggs or tucking it underneath a sliced avocado on toast. Literally any vegetable will do, from spinach, mushrooms, or tomatoes to zucchini, artichokes, sauerkraut, lentils, or lettuce.

• **They don't contain anything sweet**, **except optional whole fruit** (that is just for flavor if you enjoy it—it's not necessary). No dried fruit or fruit juices, no honey or agave or other sugars. If you've got to ask whether something is okay, it probably isn't. But remember: You can eat sweet foods the rest of the day. Just not for breakfast.

• **They contain optional starches**, such as bread or potatoes or a tortilla, for flavor, if your taste buds want them.

How to know if you're doing it right

An important rule of thumb that will tell you if your savory breakfast is working its magic on your glucose levels is if **it keeps you full for four hours**. If you have breakfast at 8 a.m., you shouldn't feel hungry until noon. That's longer than you would expect, but that's what to aim for. If you're feeling hungry before that, up the quantities. You can double or triple your breakfast recipe, or combine several breakfast options into one. Most people find that hitting this objective requires them to eat more for breakfast than they ever had before, and that's a good thing.

As you start building savory breakfasts into your life, you should feel that you don't have any more cravings in the morning, but you might still have some in the afternoon or the evening. First, don't try to resist them—eat what you are craving. Second, have a look at your lunch and dinner. Inspire yourself from the main dishes section (pages 226–51). Try to make sure that, as with breakfast, your meals are not made up exclusively of sugar or starches. That will help reduce the cravings.

Tips from the community

- Don't hesitate to eat more than you usually would at breakfast so that you hit that full-for-four-hours objective. Combining recipes also works and is quite fun.

- Write down a few recipes you want to try, and shop for several breakfasts in a row.

- Plan what your savory breakfast is going to be before you go to bed so that you know exactly what to reach for when you get up and don't get sidetracked into something sugary.

- If you miss your sweet breakfast foods, you can still have them during the rest of the day. The best time to have them is as dessert after lunch or dinner— that's when they will have the least impact on your glucose level.

Common questions from the community

What if I don't eat breakfast? There is no need to start having breakfast if you have never been in the habit of it. (But you can if you want—maybe it would be an interesting experiment?) Just make sure your first meal of the day is savory, whatever time that is.

What about coffee and tea? All good! They are absolutely fine to have during the Method. You can have them before your breakfast, during, or after, as long as you're not adding sugar or honey to them. In terms of milks, the least good option for your glucose is oat milk. Try to avoid it if you can. If you can't, that's okay.

How about sweeteners? Some sweeteners are okay if you can't do without them—pick stevia, monk fruit, or allulose. Avoid honey, sugar, maple syrup, and agave, as those create glucose spikes.

What time should I eat breakfast? Any time that works for you.

Can I have a savory breakfast that is not from one of these recipes? By all means. You can absolutely create your own savory breakfast from whatever suits you. Just make sure you follow the guidelines in "How to make a savory breakfast" on page 42.

What should I get if I'm eating out? If you're at a restaurant, remember the principles: protein, nothing sweet except whole fruit, starch for flavor. If you flick through the following recipe pages, you'll get some good ideas of what you can order when you're out.

   If you're buying breakfast at a coffee shop, get savory options, like avocado on toast, an egg muffin, or a ham and cheese sandwich, not a chocolate croissant or toast and jam.

Should I have the same breakfast every day or change it up? Whatever you prefer. In my study, half the people found one they liked and stuck to it every day, and half changed it up.

I work out in the morning. Will I have enough energy with these recipes? You can always add more food to your breakfast, including more starches and more whole fruit, if you feel that you need more of those to fuel your workout.

What if I already eat a savory breakfast? Great. You can either continue the one you like or try new ones from the recipes.

Can I adjust the recipes? Like scrambling instead of boiling the eggs or substituting almonds for walnuts or adding some more things in? Absolutely. Make them your own. As long as you aren't adding sugar to them or removing all the protein, you're good.

Can I add ingredients to the recipes, or remove some? Yes. You can modify any of them as needed to accommodate your tastes, preferences, allergies … You can add anything that is protein (meat, fish, eggs, dairy, plant protein), fat (butter, oils, avacados), fiber (whole fruit, whole vegetables, any kind of seed, any kind of nut), or starches (bread, rice, oats, potatoes). You can also remove the starches or whole fruit from the recipes. Just don't add any sugar. And remember, starches and whole fruit are there for flavor only. They should not be the center of your breakfast.

Why are there no oats recipes? Because oats do not make a good savory breakfast, unfortunately. They are mostly starch and create big glucose spikes. If you can't go without your oats, have them as a side, for flavor, along with a savory breakfast from the recipes.

Can I change the rye bread for another bread?
Yes, totally. Swap rye bread for sourdough, white bread, or gluten-free bread. Or even have potatoes or rice instead.

Is it okay to eat eggs every day? Yes. For a long time we thought that eating eggs was bad for our heart health. Now we know that's not true. Eating eggs does not increase cholesterol levels in the body, *and* cholesterol levels aren't actually that predictive of heart disease! If you want to understand more on this, pick up my first book, *Glucose Revolution*, chapter 7. But all you need to know is that switching from a sweet breakfast to a savory one *reduces* inflammation and heart disease risk.

Are carbs bad? Am I allowed to have them?
Carbohydrate ("carbs") is the word commonly used to refer to starches and sugars—that is, foods that turn to glucose when we digest them. Carbohydrates are not bad. You can absolutely eat them, and throughout this Method you will learn how to minimize their impact on your glucose. Just don't eat them on their own for breakfast. You will see during this first week of the plan that we are still including carbs (such as bread, tortillas, whole fruit) but only as a side in a meal otherwise built around protein and fat. This reduces the spikes those carbs would create. Remember that you can also eat all the carbs you want during the rest of the day.

I forgot to have a savory breakfast. Is that bad?
Not at all. It happens all the time. The Method will still work if you do it 80 percent of the time.

I'm finding it hard to give up pastries, cereal, jam, and so on at breakfast . . . Remember, you *can have* sweet foods on this Method, and the best time to eat them for your glucose is as dessert after lunch or dinner. Avoid them in your breakfast, and you will set your day up for success.

A note on cravings

I received this message from someone in the pilot experiment: "I'm feeling great, my cravings are gone, but my brain has not caught up. Does that make sense? Last night, out with my friends, I had no craving to eat the cake but I ate it anyway. When will that go away?" This is a common situation, and you may find yourself in it. Your glucose roller coaster–driven cravings will have dissipated, and you won't feel the irresistible urge to eat dessert anymore. However, the habit might still be there. It's now in your power to decide whether to eat that cake. You will have gone from a state of being overpowered by these impulses to a state in which you are in full control. My tip? Eat the cake when it's really delicious and it's your favorite type of cake. If it doesn't look that good or you're not very excited about it, pass. Remind yourself that it's so much more enjoyable to eat something you love instead of something just because it's there. As your cravings dissipate, it's important to check in with your urges; and if you find you're not actually hankering for anything, be flexible and allow yourself to update your habits. If this sounds a little abstract right now, don't worry—we will be revisiting this idea over the weeks to come.

The perfect 7-MIN EGGS

What you need:

4 eggs

+ salt and pepper

Let's start with this very simple savory breakfast recipe. The only prerequisite skill for preparing perfect 7-min eggs is a general knowledge of how to fill a pot with water. If you can turn a few handles and levers, you're golden. You can even cook the eggs in advance and take them with you to work—with a little bit of sea salt in a small piece of folded aluminum foil. Feel free to modify how many eggs you're having until they keep you full for four hours. For some people it will be two eggs; for others, six.

How to make it:

● Place a small saucepan of water on high heat and bring the water to a boil. When the water is bubbling, gently lower in the **eggs** and cook them for 7 minutes, which should be enough to gooey–hard boil them.

● Drain the water from the pan and run the eggs under cold water until they're cool enough to handle.

● Peel the eggs, then place them on a plate and cut them in half. Marvel at the perfect gooeyness!

● Season with **salt** and **pepper**, and pick them up with your fingers to eat.

Makes: 4 eggs / Prep time: until the water boils / Total cook time: 7 min
GLUTEN-FREE, VEGETARIAN

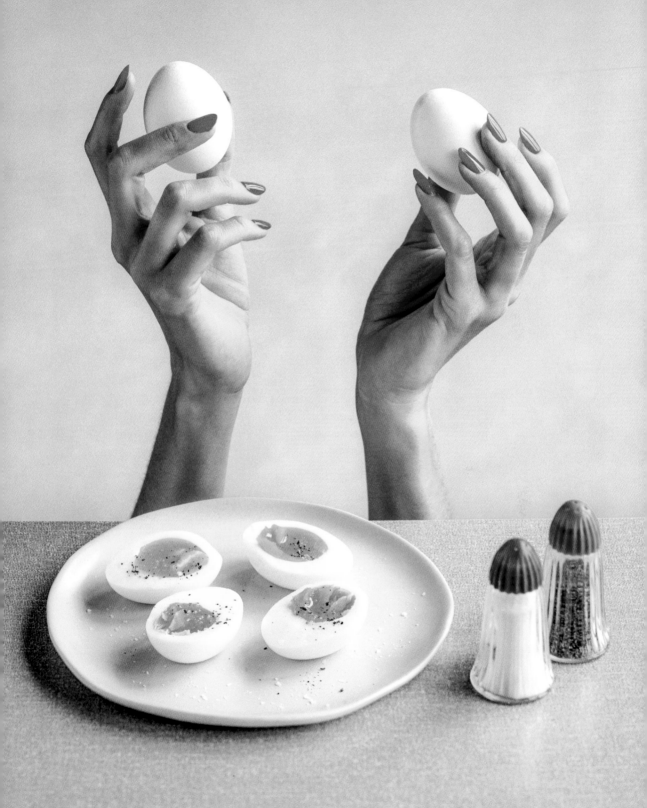

SAVORY JAM ON TOAST

What you need:

1 x 10.5-ounce/300g jar of roasted red peppers, drained and finely chopped

7 ounces/200g feta, crumbled

2 teaspoons dried oregano (optional)

sourdough or rye bread, toasted, to serve

+ ¼ cup/60ml olive oil
+ salt and pepper

A classic with a twist: we all know jam on toast, but have you met its savory cousin that keeps your glucose levels steady and leaves you feeling amazing? I can't wait for you to try it.

How to make it:

● Preheat the oven to 400°F. Place the chopped **red peppers**, crumbled **feta**, oregano (if using), and **olive oil** in a baking dish and mix them together really well. Transfer the dish to the oven and bake the feta mixture for 10 minutes, until the feta has melted and the peppers have heated through.

● Remove the dish from the oven and mix the contents together some more, then spread one third of the mixture on top of some freshly toasted **sourdough or rye bread**.

● Transfer the remaining savory jam to a jar and refrigerate for up to 2 weeks, using it as the mood takes you. It is lovely warm (just reheat in the microwave) or cold on more slices of toast.

TIP: Top the savory jam with some flaked canned tuna (drained).

Makes: 1 x 16-ounce/450g jar (enough for about 3 slices of toast)
Prep time: 6–8 min / Total cook time: 10 min
VEGETARIAN

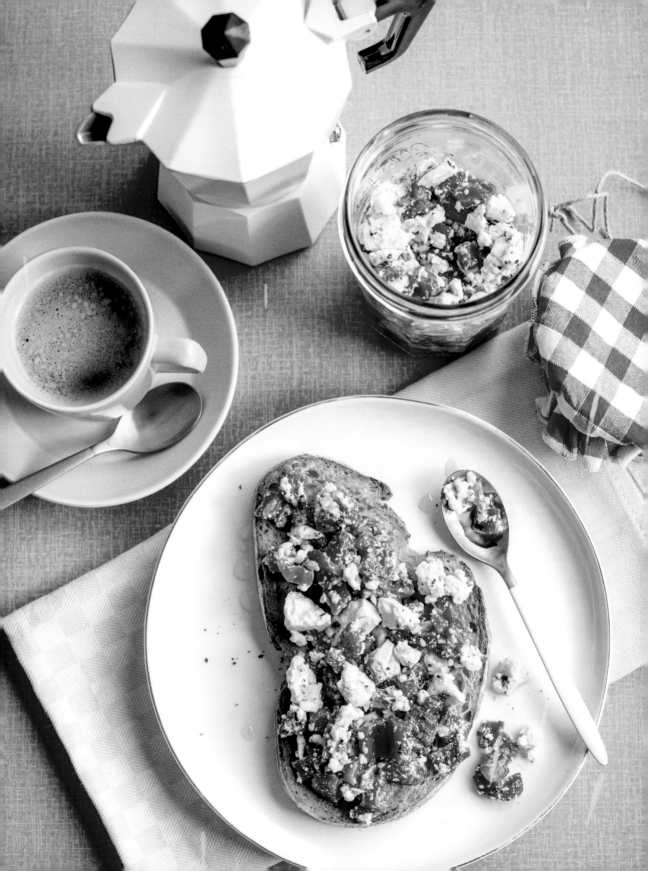

No-spike GRANOLA

What you need:

1 teaspoon coconut oil

1½ teaspoons ground cinnamon

¾ cup/100g pumpkin seeds

½ cup/50g pecan pieces

⅓ cup/50g unblanched almonds or hazelnuts (or use blanched, if you prefer)

full-fat Greek yogurt and berries, for serving

+ salt

Granola? More like graNOla. Sadly, typical granola is packed full of starch and sugar, causing a massive breakfast glucose spike. No thanks! If you're a granola lover, you don't have to totally kick it to the curb, but you do need to rework the original recipe. I've got you. This version gets its sweetness from whole fruit and uses Greek yogurt to pack it full of protein. It yields four portions, so share the extra with friends, or keep it in an airtight container and eat it for multiple mornings. Enjoy!

How to make it:

● Preheat the oven to 400°F and line a sheet pan with parchment paper. Place the **coconut oil** in a medium bowl and melt in the microwave. Stir in the **cinnamon** and a pinch of **salt**.

● Add the **pumpkin seeds, pecans,** and **almonds or hazelnuts** and toss to coat them in the cinnamon mixture. Transfer everything to the sheet pan lined with parchment paper and toast the nuts and seeds in the oven for 7 minutes.

● Remove the nuts and seeds from the oven and let them cool on the sheet pan. Once cold, transfer them to an airtight container and store them for up to 2 weeks.

● To serve, put a good dollop of **yogurt** in a bowl and top with 2–3 tablespoons of the granola and a small handful of **berries**.

Makes: 4 portions / Prep time: 4 min / Total cook time: 7 min
GLUTEN-FREE, VEGAN (without yogurt to serve)

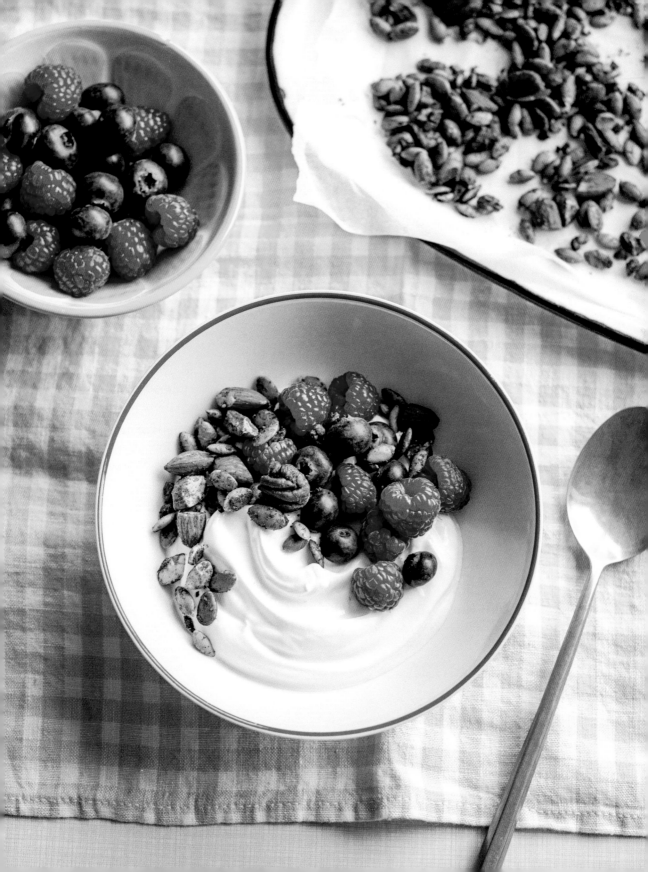

MY TWO-EGG OMELET

What you need:

a knob of butter

2 eggs, beaten

about ¾ ounce/20g feta, crumbled (you can eyeball this)

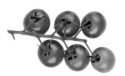

3 cherry tomatoes, halved

+ salt and pepper

Or how I like to start my day with a bang. Thin like a crêpe and bursting with flavors, this omelet is my go-to savory breakfast and is ridiculously easy to whip up. Take it to new heights by adding some arugula, and if you want to spice it up, add lots of harissa. A community favorite for a quick and efficient morning. Don't hesitate to add more eggs until this keeps you full for four hours.

How to make it:

● Place a medium nonstick frying pan on low heat and add the **butter**.

● While the butter is melting, season the beaten **eggs** with **salt** and **pepper**.

● When the butter is melted and bubbling, pour the beaten eggs into the pan, and tilt and swirl the pan to spread them out in a thin layer that covers the entire bottom. Scatter the crumbled **feta** and halved **tomatoes** over one half of the omelet, then let it cook for 1½ minutes or until set, without letting it color.

● Fold the uncovered half of the omelet over the topped half and transfer the omelet to a plate. Enjoy as a perfect start to your day.

Makes: 1 portion / Prep time: 3 min / Total cook time: 2 min
GLUTEN-FREE, VEGETARIAN

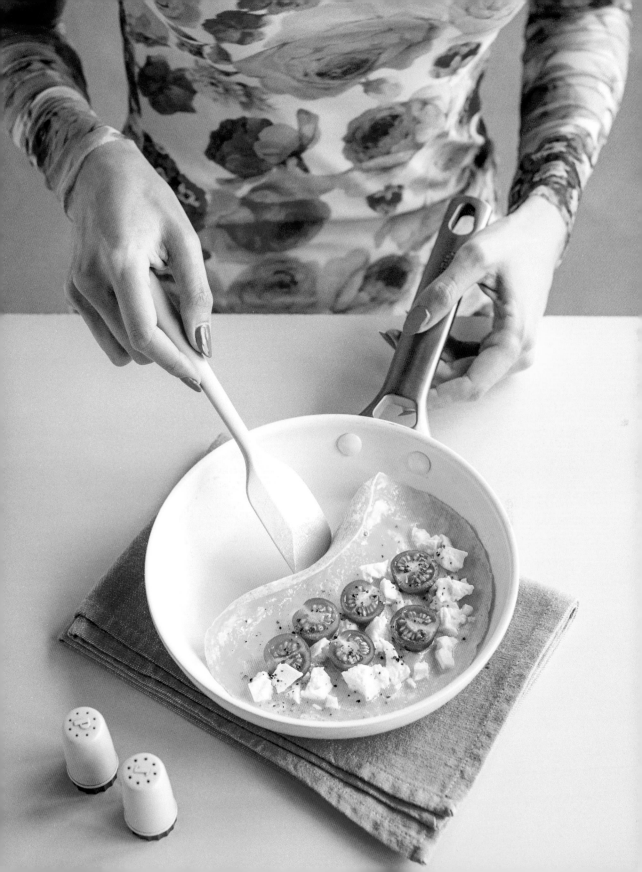

Happy HALLOUMI

What you need:

2½ ounces/70g halloumi, cut into 2 equal slices

1 garlic clove, peeled and roughly chopped

1-inch/2.5cm piece of ginger, peeled and roughly chopped

1 teaspoon garam masala or curry powder

¼ teaspoon chile powder (as hot as you like; optional)

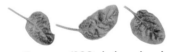

7 ounces/200g baby spinach leaves

+ olive oil
+ salt and pepper

If this halloumi makes you happy . . . clap your hands! This recipe is full of all the savory breakfast necessities: protein, fat, and fiber. As you ride into your day with steady energy and no cravings, your glucose will thank you.

How to make it:

● Heat a splash of **olive oil** in a large frying pan on medium heat and fry the sliced **halloumi** for 1 minute on each side, until golden all over. Push the halloumi to one side of the pan and lower the heat a little.

● Add a drop more olive oil to the empty side of the pan and add the chopped **garlic** and **ginger**. Fry them for 30 seconds, or until they are just starting to crisp.

● Lower the heat slightly and add the **garam masala or curry powder** and the chile powder (if using). Mix well using a wooden spoon or spatula.

● Stir the **spinach** into the garlic and spice mixture and cook for 30 seconds more, until the spinach is just starting to wilt.

● Plate the spinach and top with the halloumi. Add **salt** and **pepper** to taste before serving.

Makes: 1 portion / Prep time: 4 min / Total cook time: 4 min
GLUTEN-FREE, VEGETARIAN

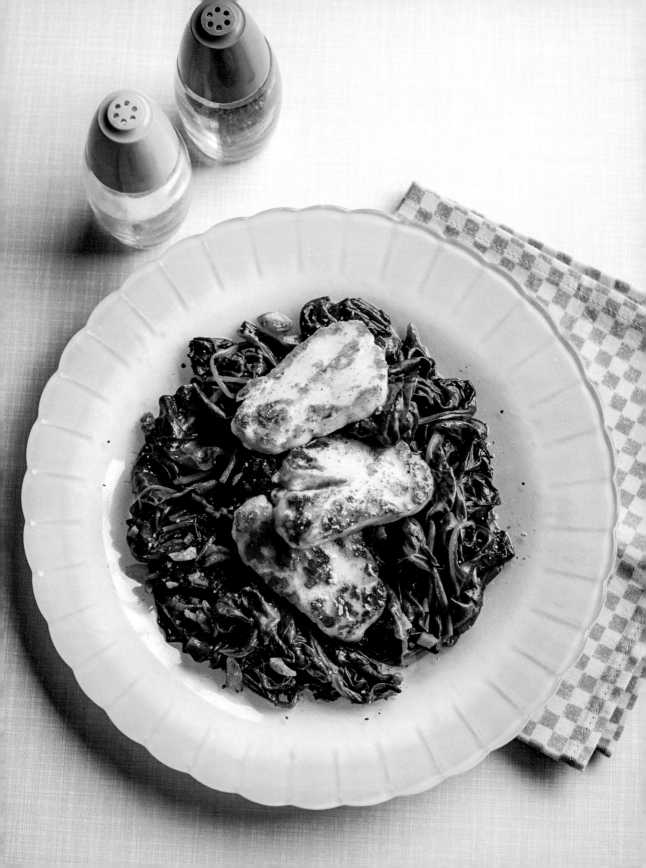

Cozy QUICHE

What you need:

butter, for greasing

1 sheet (11¼ ounces/320g) of store-bought pie dough

½ cup/150g full-fat Greek yogurt

2 whole eggs, plus 2 egg yolks

⅓ cup/60g frozen peas

2¼ ounces/60g goat cheese log, cut into 6 equal slices

1 tablespoon chopped chives

+ salt and pepper

What do a thick sweater and this fluffy quiche have in common? You've got it: they are both delightfully cozy and comforting. Make this one on a slow morning and enjoy it for the following three days—the recipe yields four perfect portions. You'll need baking beans or rice and parchment paper for "blind-baking" the pastry crust and avoiding a soggy bottom.

How to make it:

● Preheat the oven to 400°F. Generously grease an (8-inch/ 20cm-diameter and 1-inch/2.5cm-deep) nonstick cake pan that has a removable bottom with **butter**. Line the pan with the **pie dough**, pressing it gently into the corner at the bottom of the pan. Trim the overhang with a sharp knife to neaten. Crimp the edges of the dough together if you like.

● Cut out a piece of parchment paper twice the diameter of the pan, scrunch it up a little, and lay it over the pastry dough (it's going to protect the pastry from the baking beans or rice). Fill with some dried beans or rice, then transfer it to the oven and blind bake it (bake it without its filling so that your final quiche crust is nice and crisp) for 15 minutes, until lightly golden and firm.

● While the quiche crust is baking, prepare the filling. In a bowl, whisk together the **yogurt**, **whole eggs**, and **egg yolks** with a generous seasoning of **salt** and **pepper**. Stir in the **frozen peas** and set the filling aside.

● When the quiche crust is ready, remove it from the oven and discard the beans or rice and parchment paper (you can keep the beans or rice to use for blind baking another time, but don't try to eat them!). Return the quiche crust to the oven for 5 minutes, until the pastry is golden.

● Carefully pour the prepared filling into the baked quiche crust and top the filling with the slices of **goat cheese** and sprinkle with the chopped **chives**. Bake the filled quiche in the oven for 25 minutes, or until the filling is golden brown and set.

Makes: 4 generous portions / Prep time: 15 min / Total cook time: 45 min
VEGETARIAN

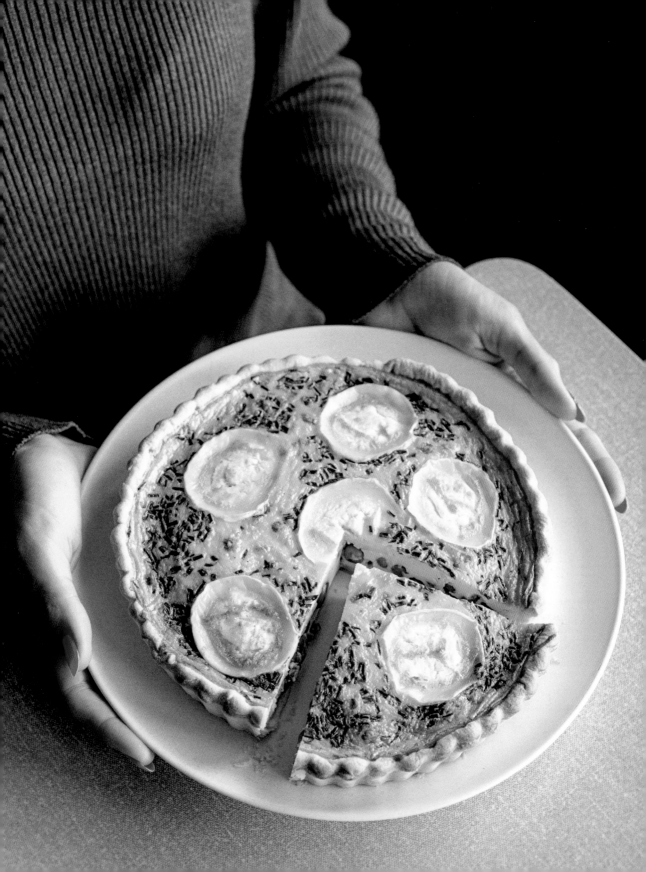

CALIFORNIA QUESADILLA

What you need:

a knob of butter

1 small skinless, boneless salmon fillet (about 4¼ ounces/120g), roughly chopped

1 6-inch flour or corn tortilla

1 tablespoon full-fat cream cheese

½ avocado, pitted and thinly sliced (save the other half for the Avocado Toast 2.0 on page 68)

a drizzle of hot sauce, such as sriracha

+ salt and pepper

Please allow me to introduce the California quesadilla, passed on to me by a friend from Los Angeles: crisp tortilla, cool cream cheese, flaky salmon, and a punch of heat. It will satisfy your glucose and your beach vacation cravings.

How to make it:

● Melt the **butter** in a medium nonstick frying pan on medium heat. Once it's bubbling, add the chopped **salmon** and cook the fish pieces for about 3 minutes, stirring from time to time.

● While the salmon is cooking, place the **tortilla** on a flat surface and spread the **cream cheese** over one half of it. Top with the **avocado** slices, then slide the salmon from the pan on top.

● Drizzle with some **hot sauce** (as much as you dare!) and season generously with **salt** and **pepper**.

● Fold the uncovered half of the tortilla over the topped half, then slide it into the frying pan. Cook it for 3 minutes, or until it's starting to turn golden and crisp. When you're ready, transfer it to a serving plate, cut it in half, and enjoy.

Makes: 1 portion / Prep time: 5 min / Total cook time: 6 min

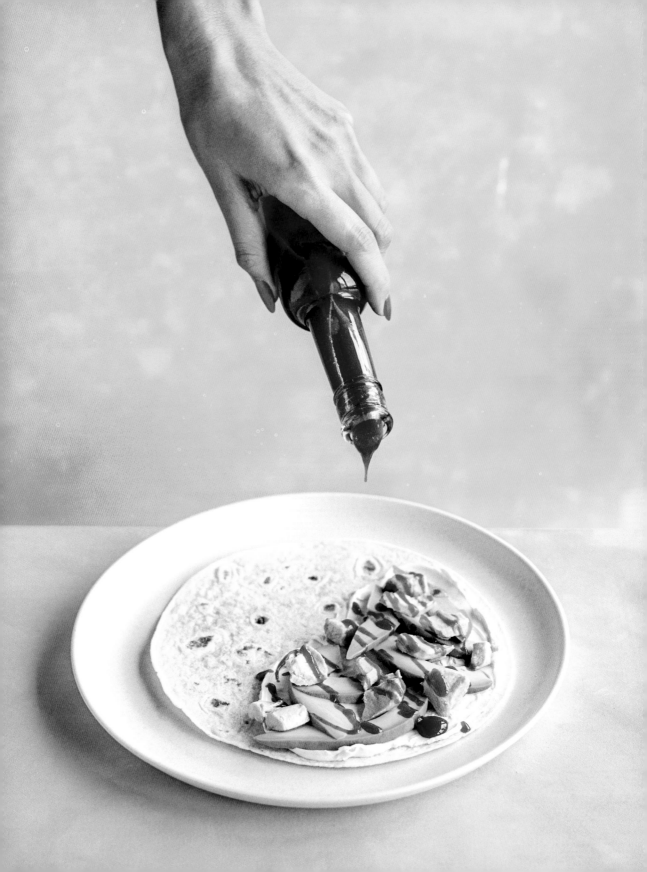

Cheeky CHICKPEA STEW

What you need:

½ onion, roughly chopped

2 garlic cloves, roughly chopped

3 tomatoes, roughly chopped

1 x 15-ounce/425g can of chickpeas, drained

½ teaspoon paprika

a dollop of full-fat Greek yogurt, to serve (optional)

+ olive oil
+ salt and pepper

Stop right there! This recipe is a winner. While most stews are time-consuming to cook, this community favorite can be whipped up in about 10 minutes with very little prep.
You could add a handful of spinach just before the end of cooking time, or serve it with a fried or poached egg on top and a slice of sourdough. You can keep it in the fridge for up to four days.

How to make it:

● Heat a splash of **olive oil** in a medium saucepan on medium heat and add the chopped **onion**. Fry for 1½ minutes, stirring occasionally, until the onion has softened, then add the chopped **garlic** and fry for 30 seconds more.

● Add the chopped **tomatoes**, **chickpeas**, **paprika**, and ⅔ cup/160ml of **water** to the pan. Increase the heat to high, cover the pan with a lid, and simmer the mixture for 7 minutes, until the tomatoes begin to break down.

● Season generously with **salt** and **pepper**, then transfer half of the stew to a bowl. Serve it just as it is or with a dollop of Greek yogurt on top, if you like.

● Allow the remaining stew to cool, then transfer it to an airtight container and refrigerate it for up to 4 days—this is your second portion for another time.

Makes: 2 portions / Prep time: 4 min / Total cook time: 10 min
GLUTEN-FREE (without bread to serve), VEGAN (without yogurt to serve)

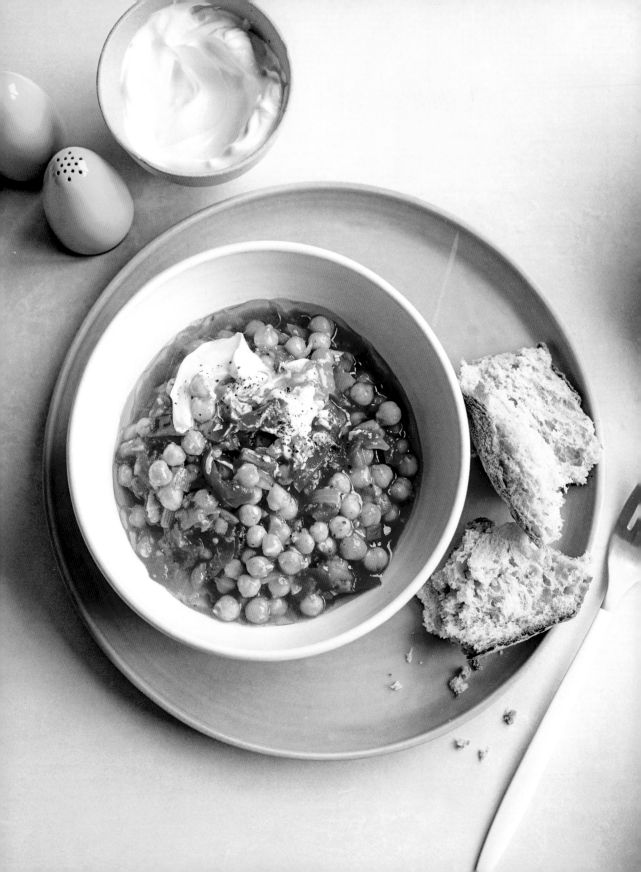

Rush-hour EGG CUPS

What you need:

a knob of butter

**3 brown button mushrooms,
finely sliced**

3 green onions, finely sliced

**1 small red bell pepper,
seeded and finely chopped**

**4 stalks Broccolini, tough
ends discarded, finely
chopped**

**6 eggs, whisked until
completely smooth**

**1¾ ounces/50g feta,
crumbled**

+ **vegetable (or other
    flavorless) oil**
+ **salt and pepper**

For those of us who live on the go . . . Make these egg cups in advance and take a couple of them with you as you head out the door in the morning. Easy to enjoy on your way to work or when you get to your desk. You'll need a six-cup silicone muffin mold to make these beauties.

How to make it:

• Preheat the oven to 400°F. Brush the cups of a six-cup silicone muffin mold with a little **vegetable oil** and set aside.

• Melt the **butter** in a medium frying pan on medium heat. Add the sliced **mushrooms**, sliced **green onions**, chopped **red bell pepper**, and chopped **Broccolini** and fry them for 4–5 minutes, until softened. Set them aside to cool a little.

• In a large bowl, generously season the whisked **eggs** with **salt** and **pepper**.

• Add the cooled vegetables and crumbled **feta** to the bowl with the eggs and stir to combine. Spoon the mixture equally into the cups of the muffin mold.

• Bake the muffins in the oven for 15–17 minutes, or until risen and set. Let the muffins cool slightly before removing them from the mold. Two muffins make a substantial breakfast, there and then. The remainder will keep in an airtight container in the fridge for up to 2 days (you can reheat them in the microwave for 20 seconds before eating, if you wish).

**Makes: 6 muffins (about 3 portions) / Prep time: 8 min
Total cook time: 22 min
GLUTEN-FREE, VEGETARIAN**

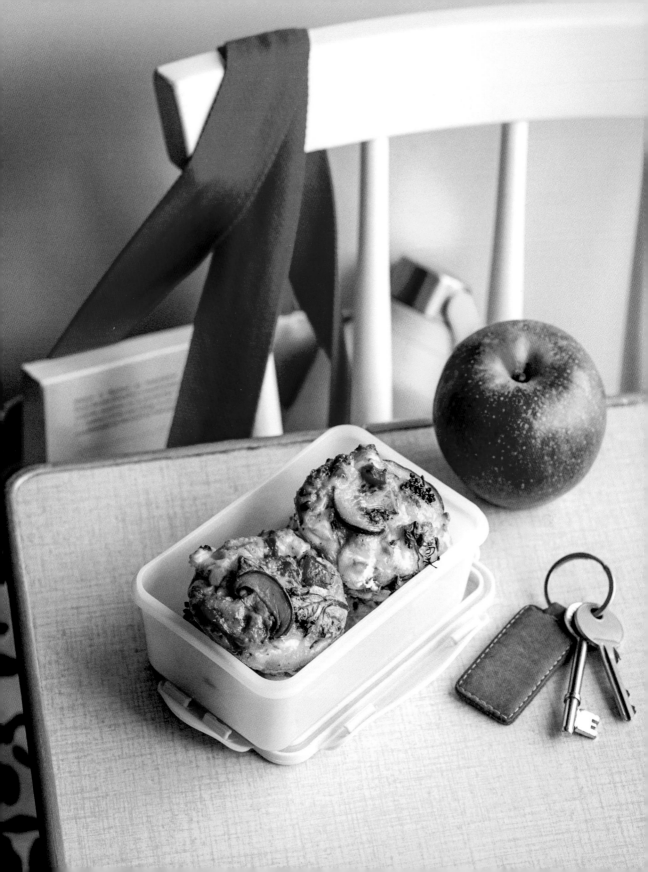

TODAY *I'm fancy* SALMON TOAST

What you need:

1 slice of rye bread

1 heaping tablespoon of full-fat cream cheese

1 slice of smoked salmon, cut in half

2 teaspoons capers, drained

a wedge of lemon, for squeezing

In this first week of the Glucose Goddess Method, you are becoming a Goddess, God, or Nonbinary Deity. Deities can get fancy, and it's for those days that this fancy salmon toast was created. Up the salmon quantity until it keeps you full for four hours, and scatter over a few salad leaves to serve, if you like.

How to make it:

● Toast the slice of **rye bread**. Spread the **cream cheese** evenly over the toast and top with the **salmon** and **capers**. Serve with the **lemon** wedge for squeezing.

Makes: 1 portion / Prep time: 7 min

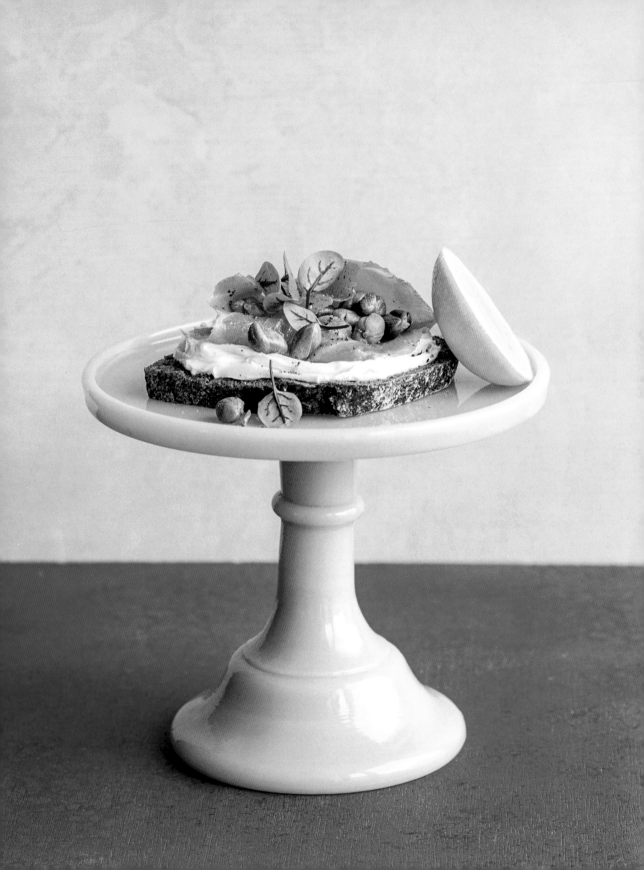

SPINACH AND SAUSAGE
sitting in a tree

What you need:

2 good-quality breakfast
sausages (about
2¼ ounces/60g each),
cut into ½-inch/1cm pieces

2 garlic cloves, roughly
chopped

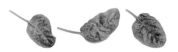

7 ounces/200g spinach
leaves

+ 1 tablespoon olive oil

Spinach leaves and sausages sitting in a tree, K-I-S-S-I-N-G.
First comes sausage, then come garlic and spinach, then
comes steady glucose levels.

How to make it:

● Heat the **olive oil** in a medium frying pan on medium heat. Add
the **sausage** pieces and fry them for 5 minutes, turning them
regularly, until they are golden brown all over. Transfer sausage
pieces to a plate and cover with foil, to keep warm.

● Add the chopped **garlic** to the fat left in the pan and fry it
for about 30 seconds to soften, then add the **spinach**. Stir
to combine, and cook the spinach until it's heated through
and wilted.

● Transfer the spinach to a serving plate, top with the sausage
pieces, and serve.

Makes: 1 portion / Prep time: 10 min / Total cook time: 7 min
GLUTEN-FREE

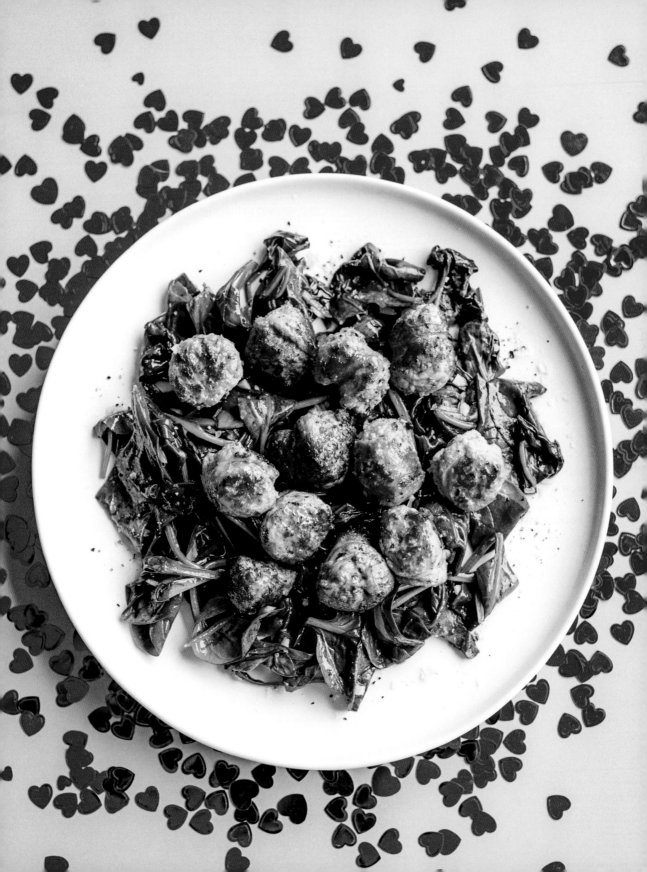

AVOCADO TOAST 2.0

What you need:

½ avocado, pitted

1 teaspoon harissa paste

1 slice of rye or sourdough bread

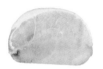

2 slices of smoked ham

a squeeze of lemon juice (optional)

+ salt and pepper

The little problem with most avocado toasts (no offense, dear avocado toasts) is that they don't contain any protein. And you know what that means: it's not a winning savory breakfast. So here's the thing—swooping in between the bread and the avocado, our glucose hero: ham! If you're not a ham person you can add cheese, eggs, tofu, or any other protein of your choice.

How to make it:

● Place the **avocado** flesh and **harissa paste** in a bowl and roughly mash them together with the back of a fork. Season the mixture with **salt** and **pepper**.

● Toast the slice of **rye or sourdough bread** and place it on a serving plate, then lay both **ham** slices on top. Top with the smashed avocado mixture.

● Squeeze a little **lemon juice** over it, if you wish, and serve.

Makes: 1 portion / Prep time: 7 min

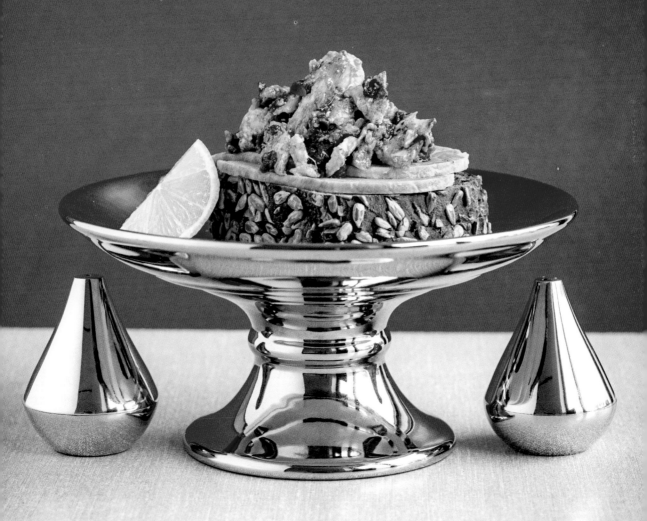

PROSCIUTTO. RICOTTA. FIGS.
Chef's kiss.

What you need:

3 tablespoons ricotta

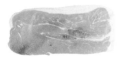

**3 slices of prosciutto
(smoked, if you can find it)**

1 fresh fig, cut into 6 wedges

**+ salt and pepper
+ olive oil, for drizzling**

A meal this decadent and this good for your glucose feels almost illegal. The prosciutto and ricotta pack a big punch of protein, and the fig is your whole fruit for taste. Make sure the fig is fresh, not dried. You can replace it with any other whole fruit (for example, a peach), and the ricotta with any other cheese (burrata and mozzarella being great contenders). And here's another idea: throw a few sliced almonds, pecan pieces, or chopped hazelnuts on top. Dreamy and steady.

How to make it:

● Place the **ricotta** in a bowl with a generous pinch of **salt** and **pepper**. Using a fork, mix the ricotta until it is smooth, then spoon it onto a serving plate.

● Top the cheese with the **prosciutto** slices and **fig** wedges, drizzle everything with **olive oil**, and grind some more pepper on top, then serve.

Makes: 1 portion / Prep time: 5 min
GLUTEN-FREE

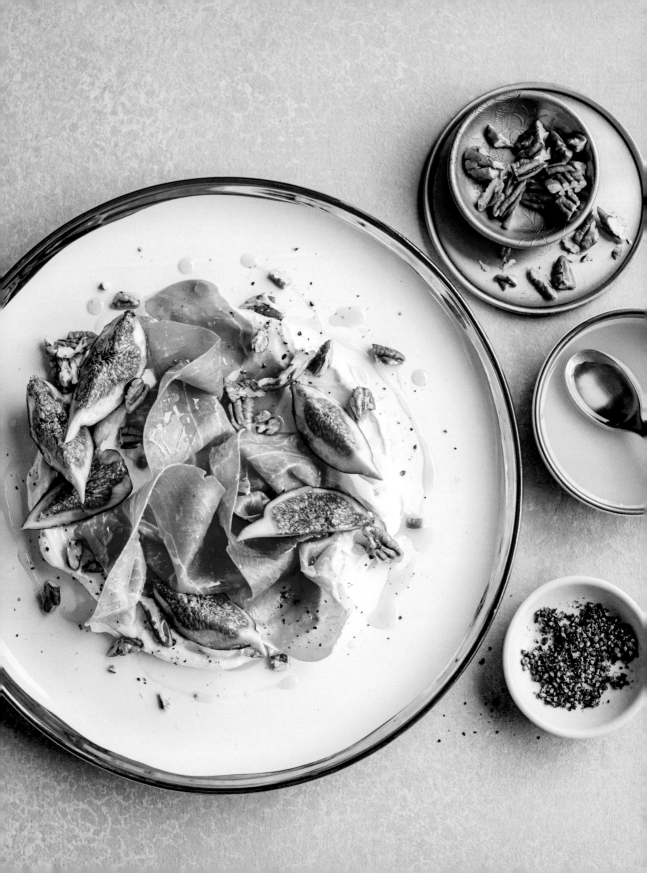

ONE-DISH DELISH

What you need:

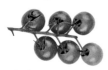

10 cherry tomatoes, halved

5 brown button mushrooms, sliced

one-quarter of 1 x 15-ounce/425g can of chickpeas, drained

1 tablespoon Worcestershire sauce

2 slices of bacon, each cut into 3 pieces

1 egg
crusty bread, to serve

+ 1 tablespoon olive oil
+ salt and pepper

This delish one-dish meal was born of the philosophy that savory breakfasts should be light on dish duty but heavy on flavor. Now nothing can keep you from the savory breakfast of your dreams. Add a toasted slice of your favorite bread to this for fun.

How to make it:

● Preheat the oven to 425°F. Place the **tomato** halves, **mushroom** slices, and **chickpeas** into a small baking dish or skillet (you're looking for a snug fit) and drizzle with the **Worcestershire sauce** and **olive oil**. Transfer the dish to the oven and bake the mixture for 5 minutes.

● Remove the dish and arrange the **bacon** pieces on top, then return everything to the oven for 10 minutes, until the bacon is cooked through and crispy at the edges.

● Remove the dish once more, crack in the **egg**, then return it to the oven and cook the egg for 6–8 minutes, until the white is set and the yolk is still a little runny. Season with salt and pepper and serve with some crusty bread to mop up the delicious juices.

Makes: 1 portion / Prep time: 5 min / Total cook time: 23 min
GLUTEN-FREE (without bread to serve)

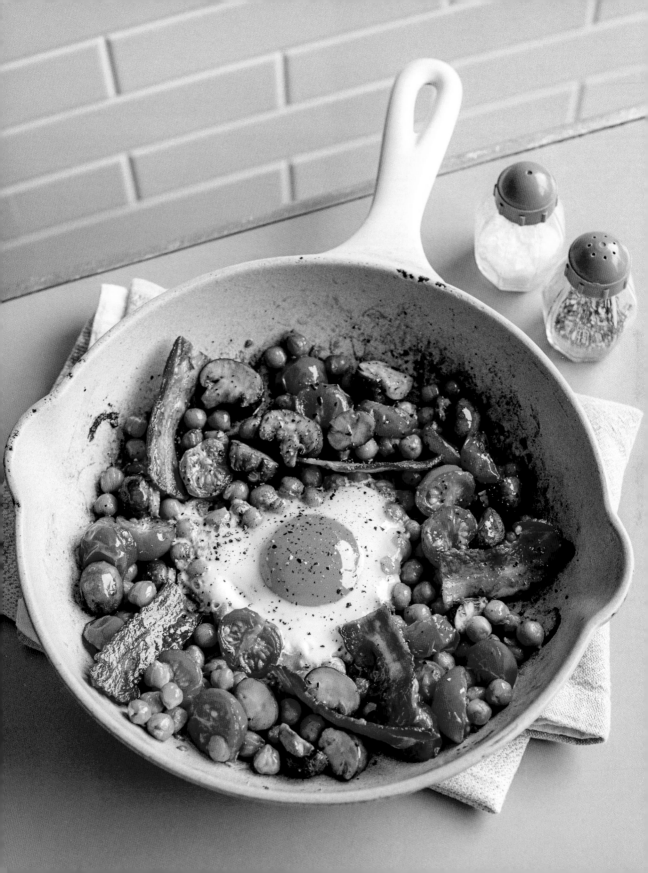

TOAST PARTY

What you need:

3 slices of dark rye bread

1 slice of smoked trout

2 tablespoons soft goat cheese

1 heaping tablespoon basil pesto

+ salt and pepper

Good news! I'm throwing a party and everyone is invited. Everyone, that is, except for naked toast. Toast is not to be shunned from our savory breakfasts, as long as it's there for flavor and you dress it up in its best party dresses: protein, fat, or fiber.

How to make it:

● Toast the slices of **rye bread** and top each with either the **smoked trout**, **goat cheese**, or **basil pesto** (one topping per piece).

● Cut each slice in half, season with **salt** and **pepper**, and serve.

Makes: 1 portion / Prep time: 10 min

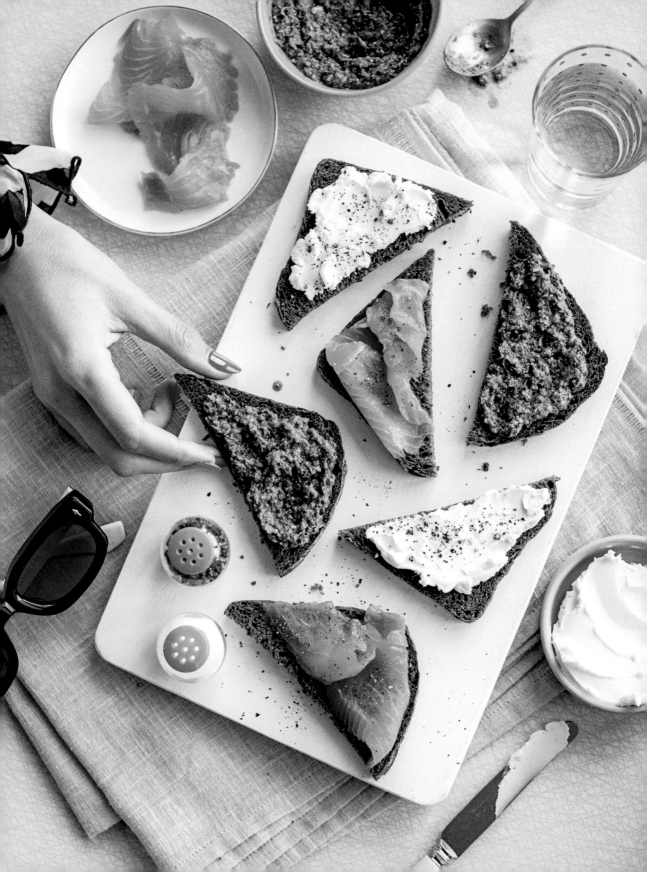

AN APPLE
with some clothes on

What you need:

1 apple (about 3¼ ounces/ 90g), sliced into rounds (there's no need to core it)

juice of ¼ lemon

1½ ounces/40g Cheddar, sliced

a small handful of walnut halves or pieces

Whole fruits are a very welcome addition to a savory breakfast, as long as they are there for taste and as long as they are accompanied by protein and fat. Basically, whole fruits should not go out naked. So here is an apple with some clothes on: protein and fat from the Cheddar and walnuts! Get ready for tart, crunchy, bitey mouthfuls.

How to make it:

● Dress the sliced **apple** with the **lemon juice** to prevent it from browning.

● Arrange the apple slices on a plate, add the **Cheddar** slices, and scatter the **walnuts**, then serve.

Makes: 1 portion / Prep time: 5 min
GLUTEN-FREE, VEGETARIAN

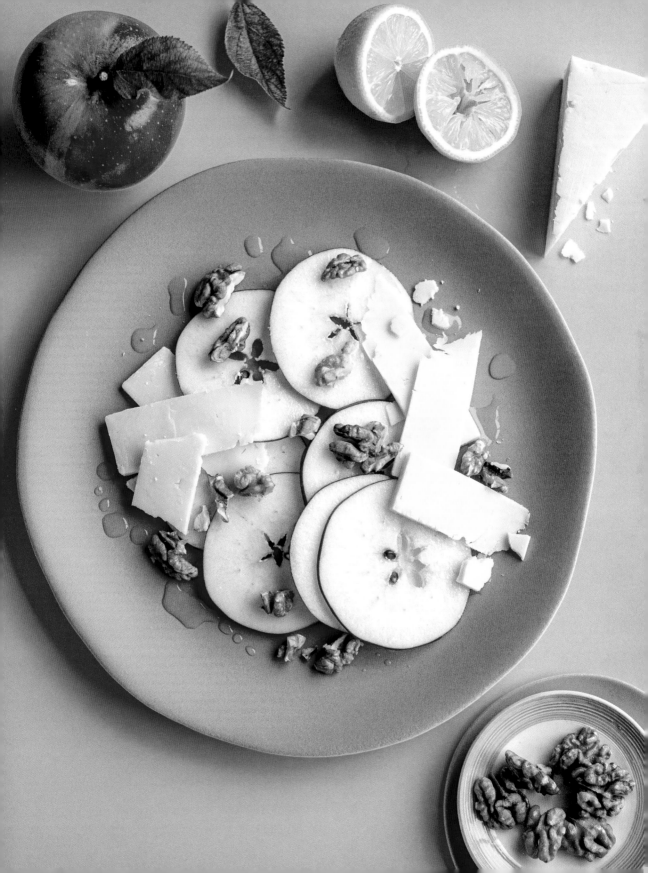

TOMATO TOAST

What you need:

1 slice of sourdough bread

a small handful of arugula

½ ball of burrata (use the other half for the Fiber-First Garden Plate on page 92)

3 sun-dried tomatoes in oil, drained and cut in half

1 heaping teaspoon good-quality basil pesto

+ ½ tablespoon olive oil
+ salt and pepper

A variation on the avocado toast . . . how about a tomato toast? (At Glucose Goddess we are big fans of alliteration.) Tasty tomato on toasted sourdough topped with terrific burrata and tangy pesto.

How to make it:

● Toast the slice of **sourdough bread**, place it on a plate, and drizzle with the **olive oil**.

● Top with the **arugula**, **burrata**, and halved **sun-dried tomatoes** and drizzle with the **basil pesto**. Season with **salt** and **pepper** and eat immediately.

Makes: 1 portion / Prep time: 5 min
VEGETARIAN

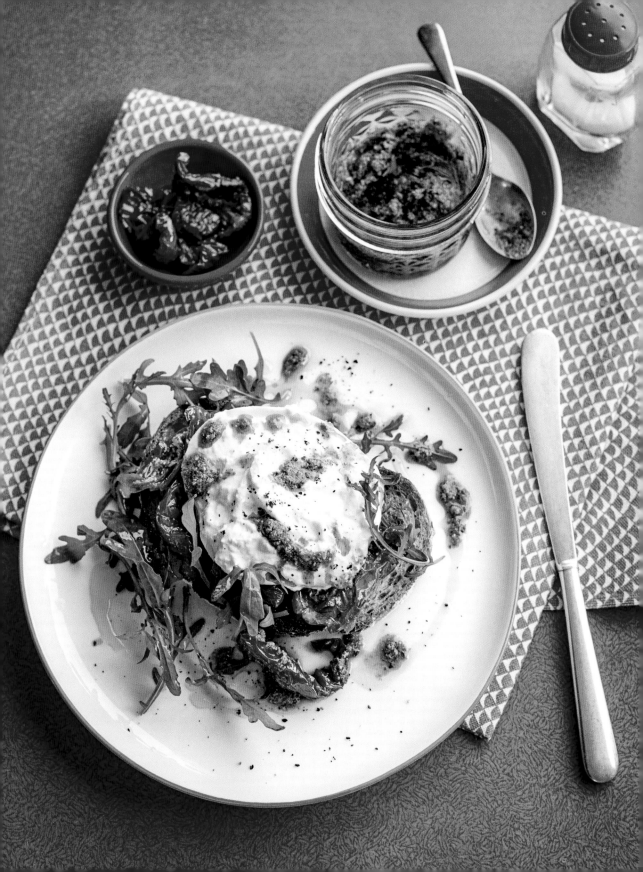

SAVORY SMOOTHIE

What you need:

2 scoops of protein powder (I recommend whey protein powder, or pea protein powder if you are vegan, but use whatever you prefer)

1 teaspoon flaxseed oil

2 teaspoons ground flaxseeds

3½ ounces/100g frozen fruit, such as blueberries (about ⅔ cup)

3 tablespoons nut butter or ¼ cup/30g nuts

Not your regular glucose-spiking fruit smoothie . . . I worked some Glucose Goddess magic on this protein-, fat-, and fiber-packed version that passes the savory test with flying colors. If you want to create your own savory smoothie, build it around protein, and add fat and fiber, and fruit for taste.

How to make it:

● Place **all of the ingredients** in a blender with 7 tablespoons/100ml of **water** and blitz until smooth. Pour into a glass, and serve.

Makes: 1 portion / Prep time: 5 min
GLUTEN-FREE, VEGAN

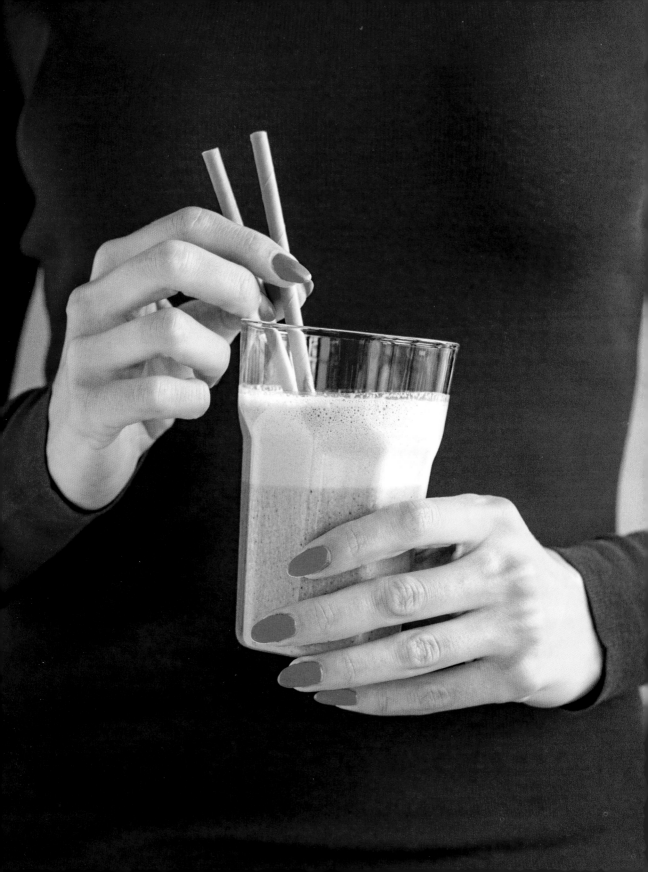

BREAKFAST ICE CREAM

What you need:

6 tablespoons/100g full-fat Greek yogurt

1 tablespoon nut butter

⅓ cup/50g frozen mixed berries

Ice cream for breakfast? Is there really any explanation needed as to why this is an amazing way to kick-start the day? This glucose-friendly version of everyone's favorite dessert features Greek yogurt, creamy nut butter, and berries. A delight.

How to make it:

● In a bowl, mix the **yogurt** and **nut butter** together until smooth.

● Stir in the **frozen mixed berries** and let the mixture settle for 2–3 minutes before eating.

Makes: 1 portion / Prep time: 5 min
GLUTEN-FREE, VEGETARIAN

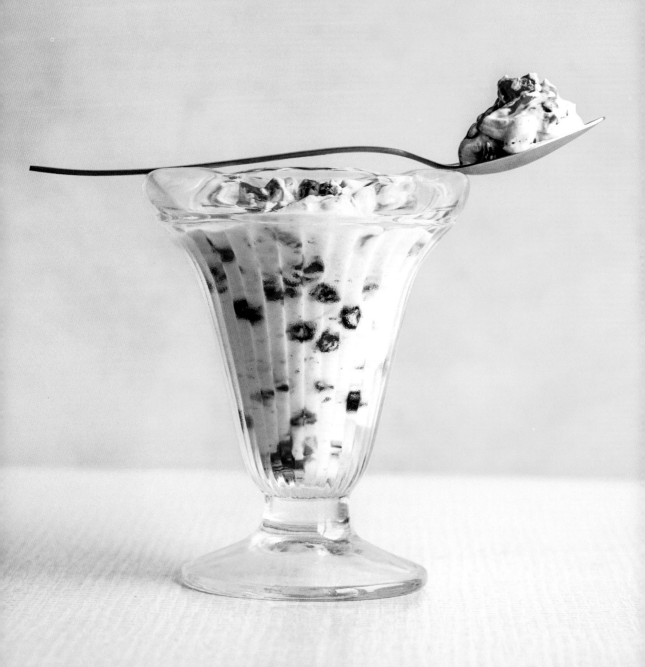

A PEACH
with some clothes on

What you need:

**3 heaping tablespoons
full-fat Greek yogurt**

**1 ripe peach, pitted and
cut into wedges**

**2 tablespoons good-quality
light tahini (good-quality
tahini will be liquidy, which is
what you want here)**

+ a pinch of sea salt

Peaches called—they were jealous that apples got some clothes to lower their glucose spike (page 76) and they didn't. So we went shopping for some protein-and-fat outfits (the yogurt and tahini), and peaches entered the ranks of our savory breakfast recipes.

How to make it:

● Place the **yogurt** and **peach** wedges in a serving bowl, drizzle with the **tahini**, sprinkle with the **sea salt**, and serve.

TIP: A few spoonfuls of No-Spike Granola (page 50) are lovely sprinkled over the top.

Makes: 1 portion / Prep time: 5 min
GLUTEN-FREE, VEGETARIAN

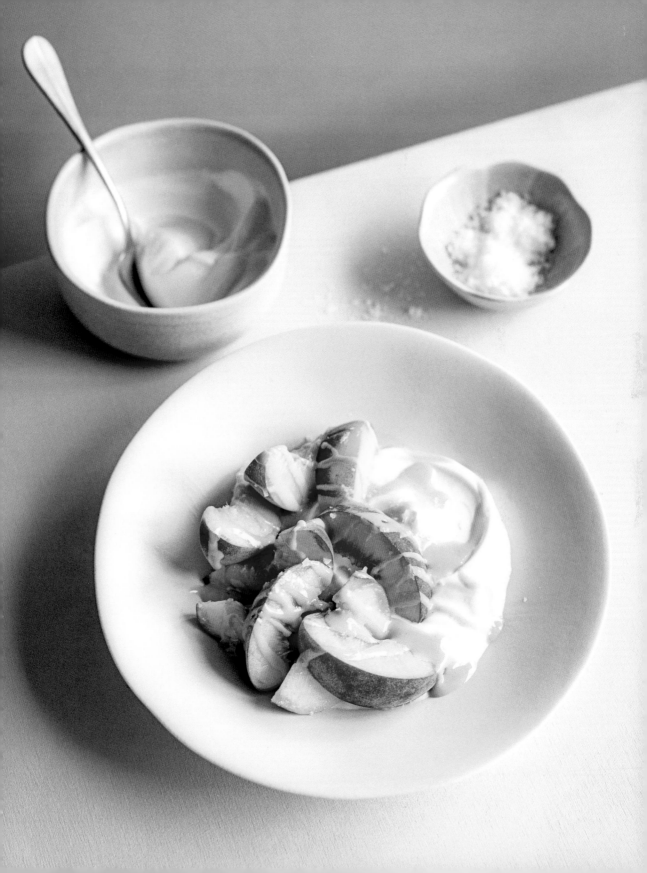

AVOCADO ACCIDENT

What you need:

½ avocado, pitted and sliced

juice of ¼ lemon

3 tablespoons hummus

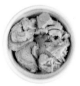

half of 1 x 5-ounce/140g can
of tuna in olive oil, drained

1 tablespoon seeds (such as
pumpkin or sunflower) and/
or nuts (such as walnuts)

+ 1 tablespoon olive oil
+ salt and pepper

Or how putting together random ingredients from my fridge turned into a classic breakfast recipe. A happy accident that has become a community favorite.

How to make it:

● Dress the sliced **avocado** with the **lemon juice** to prevent it from browning.

● Spoon the **hummus** onto a serving plate and arrange the avocado slices on top.

● Top the avocado with the drained **tuna** and the **seeds and/or nuts** and drizzle with the **olive oil**. Season with **salt** and **pepper**, and serve.

Makes: 1 portion / Prep time: 5 min
GLUTEN-FREE

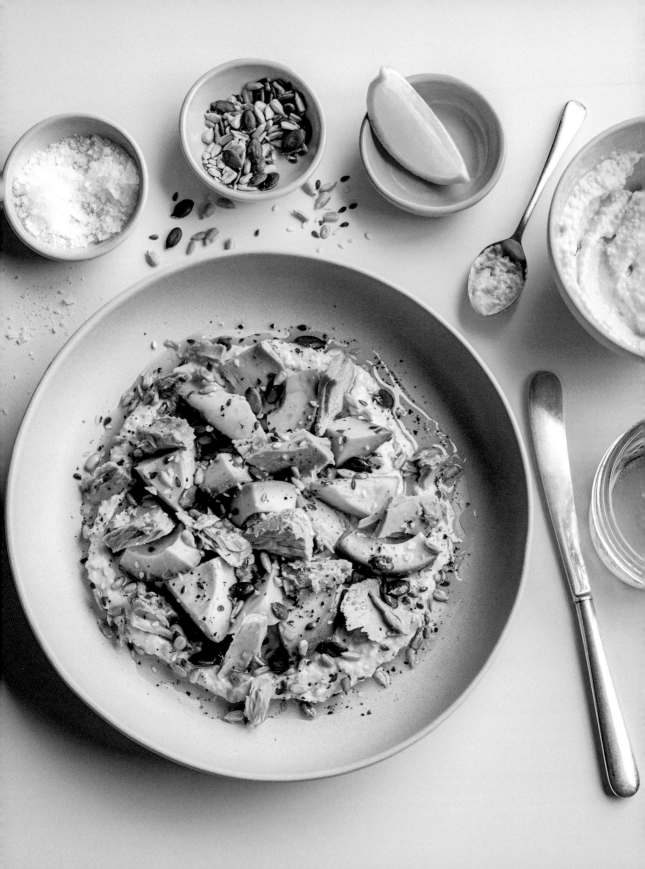

BREAKFAST SALAD

What you need:

4½ ounces/125g seeded
watermelon, rind trimmed,
roughly chopped into cubes

8 radishes, trimmed and
sliced

2¼ ounces/60g feta,
crumbled

3–4 mint sprigs, leaves
picked from the stem and
roughly chopped

2 tablespoons pumpkin
seeds

a squeeze of lime juice

+ 1 tablespoon olive oil

This easy, throw-it-together savory breakfast tastes like summertime in a bowl. The sweet watermelon against the biting flavor of mint, paired with the dueling textures of feta and nuts make this a dreamy glucose-steadying breakfast. A perfect option for when your heart says holiday.

How to make it:

● Arrange the chopped **watermelon**, sliced **radishes**, crumbled **feta**, and chopped **mint leaves** in a bowl. Sprinkle with the **pumpkin seeds** and drizzle with the **lime juice** and **olive oil**.

Makes: 1 portion / Prep time: 5 min
GLUTEN-FREE, VEGETARIAN

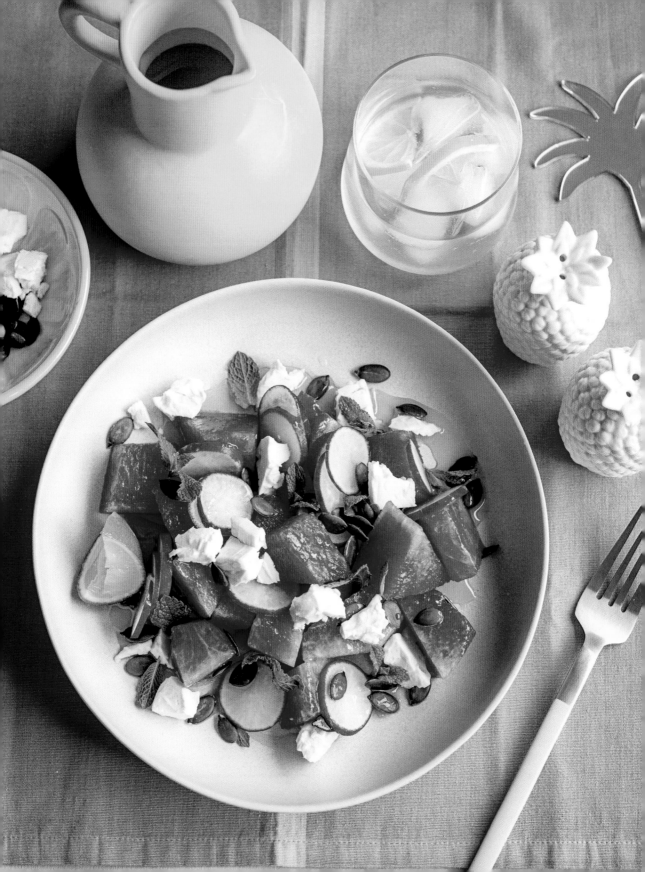

CHILE SARDINES

What you need:

½ avocado, pitted and sliced

juice of ¼ lemon

1 x 4.2-ounce/120g can of sardines in olive oil, drained

a small handful of arugula

1 tablespoon chile oil (see Tip)

+ salt and pepper

Okay, you've seen avocado in breakfast recipes before. But adding sardines and chile oil takes it from "Been there, done that" to "Where has this been all my life?" Serve these ingredients on a piece of toast for an original dish that's sure to set your glucose on a steady path for the whole day.

How to make it:

● Dress the sliced **avocado** with the **lemon juice** to prevent it from browning.

● Arrange the drained **sardines** with the **arugula** on a serving plate.

● Drizzle **chile oil** all over, season with **salt** and **pepper**, and serve.

TIP: To make your own chile oil, heat 1 tablespoon olive oil in a small saucepan along with about ¼ teaspoon chile powder (any strength you like) or ½ teaspoon chile flakes. When it starts to bubble, remove the pan from the heat and let the oil cool. Once it's cooled to room temperature, it's ready to use.

Makes: 1 portion / Prep time: 5 min

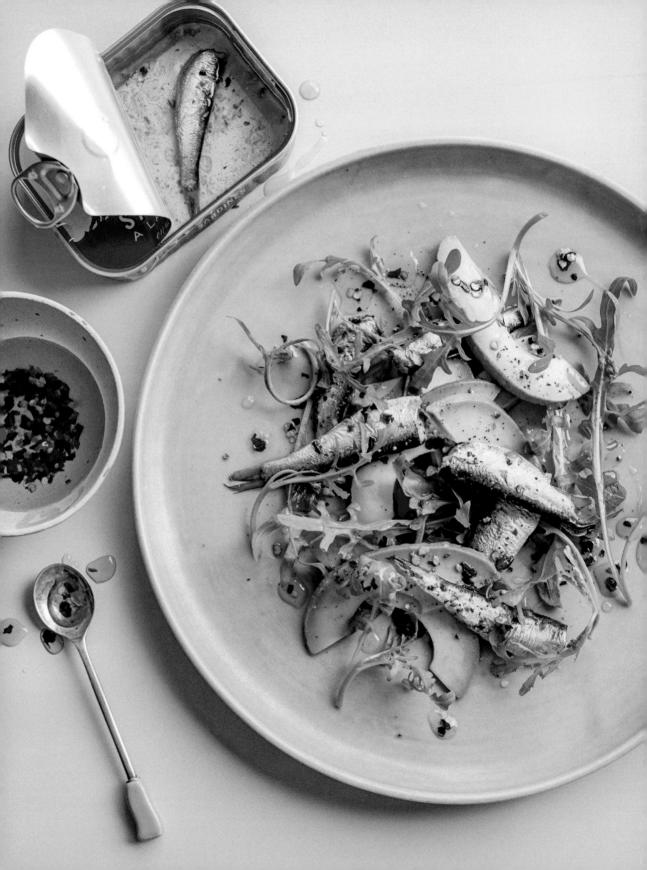

Fiber-First GARDEN PLATE

What you need:

½ ball of burrata (reserve the other half for the Tomato Toast on page 78)

1 small peach, pitted and sliced

a small handful of arugula

2 tablespoons chopped pecans

+ 1 tablespoon olive oil
+ salt and pepper

If you want to be extra helpful to your glucose, eat the arugula in this dish first. When we eat vegetables at the beginning of the meal, we reduce the glucose spike of the rest of the meal. Might this be a little preview of what's to come in Week 3? Perhaps!

How to make it:

● Arrange the **burrata**, **peach** slices, **arugula**, and **pecans** in a serving bowl and drizzle them with the **olive oil**. Season with **salt** and **pepper**, and serve.

Makes: 1 portion / Prep time: 5 min
GLUTEN-FREE, VEGETARIAN

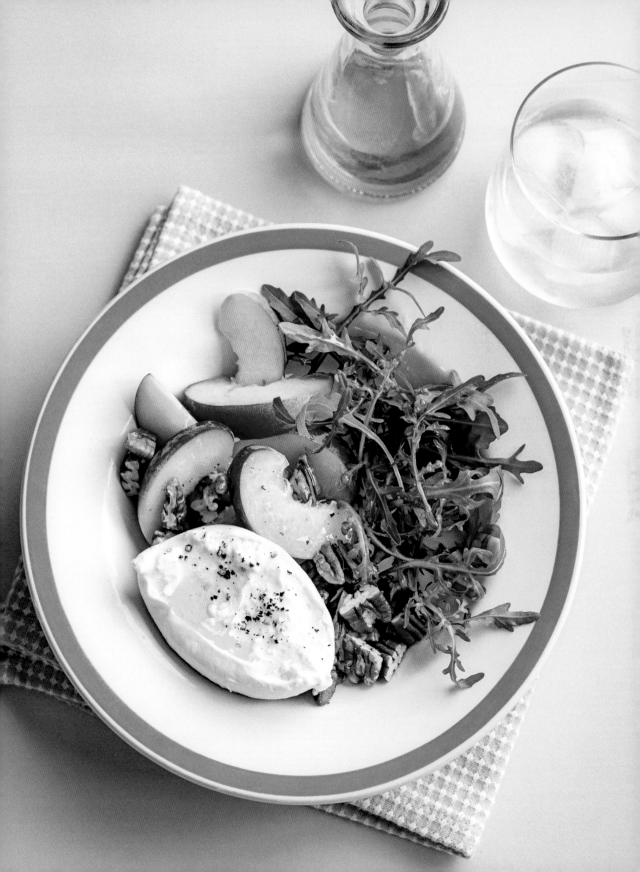

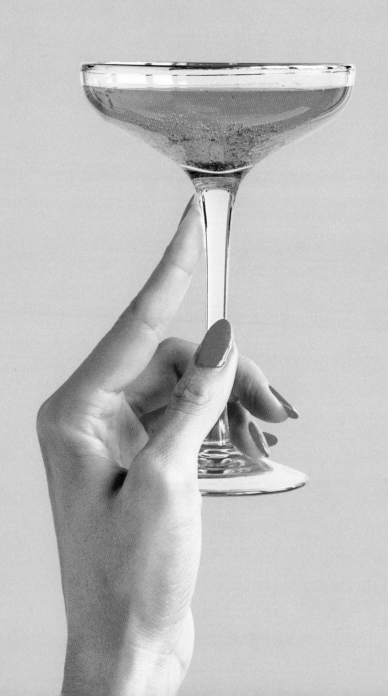

VINEGAR

Oh my gosh! Look at you! You're glowing. It must be the steady glucose levels.

TESTIMONIALS FROM THE COMMUNITY

"I feel so good with the vinegar in my diet. I honestly feel that my cravings are not there anymore."

"Day 13: Last night I slept six hours straight!! First time in years."

"I don't have any more digestive problems . . . no more pain and no more gas—feeling lighter and less swollen."

"This week I was able to go one day without eating late with no problem. This has never happened in my whole life. I am 45 years old and I am Mexican. When I was growing up, we ate dinner and then went to sleep. It is my biggest obstacle to healing and it is actually getting healed!"

"I can go so long without being hungry—like four to five and a half hours. My body feels nourished. It's super annoying being hungry every three hours. The vinegar has been a GAME CHANGER for long-lasting satiety."

"My belly is flatter even though I didn't want to lose weight. Until now, I have always had a little bloated belly."

"I'm feeling great; I think about my cravings only when I open kitchen cabinets and find snacks I have forgotten about. I think this will lead to weight loss in the long run."

"My psoriasis spots are less red and flaky."

"I've improved my mood swings. I notice I no longer go from 0 to 100 in one second. I'm more calm. That's a lot for me! (Three kids: 8, 5, and 2 years hahahaha.)"

"My energy level and reduction of cravings—spectacular."

"I'm in such a good mood it's ridiculous."

"No more sugar cravings! Never thought that I could survive a day without chocolate."

"For the first time in my life I'm really motivated. I've lost almost five pounds and my energy levels are way better!!! I'm so happy—still 17 pounds to go."

"I used to feel sleepy after lunch but it's all gone now. I've replaced my after-lunch nap with a book-reading session."

"My energy levels have improved a lot. . . . I went back to old habits (sweet breakfast and no vinegar) for three days because I was sick but I immediately felt the difference: nausea came back and I felt hungry all the time."

"I'm dealing with an intense family situation, and normally my weight would shoot up with the stress. But to my surprise, I'm actually losing weight during this second week. I'm really enjoying the vinegar in my water."

"The lack of hunger is outstanding. I used to be hungry all day, and now I'm fine doing three meals a day. I have also had the energy to do small exercise routines, which I never used to be in the mood for."

"I feel more grounded when I am choosing what I will eat—it's letting me choose the food properly. Just a BIG thank-you for this Method!"

"Week 2: My skin is clearer, I feel more connected to my body, and I listen to my body more, which is fantastic."

"Cravings have reduced, and I spend less time and mental energy thinking about food. It is freeing! No decrease in bloating and IBS-C symptoms but I feel generally better!"

"I feel less guilty about eating sweet stuff. Before finding this Method, I would berate myself for having sweet stuff at any time. With the knowledge I have now, I know I can have some if I want to and not feel bad about it!"

"No cravings (my husband works for a chocolate company and we always have products at home—cravings disappeared!). THANK YOU!"

"I feel like my gut health has improved. I feel like I no longer have hypoglycemia, something I've had my whole life."

"I have type 2 diabetes. Mentally, I am so much more motivated because I have energy and feel so much more positive. Physically, my blood sugar has not been climbing as high post-meals and I have been able to reduce the amount of insulin I need, too. This has had a massive impact on my moods. I'm less irritable. I have so much more energy!"

Your objective for Week 2

Your objective during Week 2 is to continue your savory breakfasts (we will continue them all the way to the end of the Method) and to start deploying the vinegar hack. Like a secret agent on a mission, you can use this hack tactically—have your vinegar when it is most advantageous for you and will most effectively slash your glucose spikes.

Your objective is to **consume one tablespoon of vinegar each day**. You will discover all sorts of different ways you can do this (drinking, drizzling, pickling . . .) in the recipes.

You can have your vinegar at any time during the day. Most people will have the entire tablespoon of vinegar in the morning, before their savory breakfast, because they find it easier to remember to do it then. But you can also sip it in small amounts during the course of the day until you get to a total of one tablespoon.

While any time is fine, the most powerful moment to have your vinegar is **before eating something sweet** (like a sugary snack, cookie, bar of chocolate, dessert) or **before eating something starchy** (pasta, bread, potatoes, rice), because it will significantly reduce the glucose spike of that sweet or starchy food (remember, sweet and starchy foods are the foods that are most likely to create spikes, because they break down into glucose as we digest them). If you have your vinegar before those foods, you'll be able to enjoy them with less likelihood of starting a cravings roller coaster.

And when it comes to timing it before a meal, **10 minutes before is optimal**. But again, there is flexibility—if you drink your vinegar 30 minutes before your meal, or during your meal, it will also have an impact.

So it's up to you to decide when to drink your vinegar—you may prefer the morning habit, or perhaps you will save it for before a starchy meal or a sweet snack. As long as you get the one tablespoon a day somehow, you're completing the hack.

And that's it! Eat your savory breakfast, take your vinegar, and you can continue going about your day as you wish.

Try to notice if you feel less tired, and if your cravings decrease. These are all short-term signs that your glucose is steadying.

The science

Scientists have found that vinegar (it doesn't matter which type) contains a powerful component called *acetic acid.* When we give acetic acid to our body, a few mind-blowing things happen: First, it slows down the rate at which our digestive enzymes break down sugars and starches into glucose. This is good, because as this process slows down, glucose molecules hit our system more softly, leading to a smaller spike. Second, once acetic acid gets into the bloodstream, it penetrates our muscles. There it encourages our muscles to soak up glucose molecules that are floating around and to store them for our next exercise.

These two factors—glucose being released into the body more slowly and our muscles taking it up more quickly—mean that there is less free-flowing glucose present. One tablespoon of vinegar before a meal can reduce the glucose spike of that meal **by up to 30 percent**, and the insulin spike **by up to 20 percent**—thereby reducing inflammation, slowing down aging, increasing energy, balancing our hormones, and helping our brain.

What's more, acetic acid not only reduces the amount of insulin present—which helps us get back into fat-burning mode—it also has a remarkable effect on our DNA. It tells our DNA to reprogram slightly so that our mitochondria burn more fat. A study found that when people added vinegar before their meals for three months, they reduced their visceral fat, waist and hip measurements, and triglyceride levels.

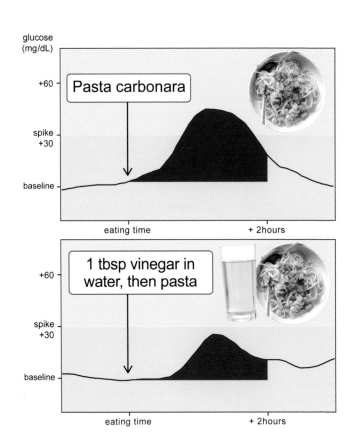

Vinegar: the very powerful Week 2 hack

How to make your own vinegar hack

All you need is one tablespoon of the vinegar of your choice—apple cider vinegar and white vinegar are the most popular vinegars to drink—and a *vehicle* to get it into your body. The vehicle can be a drink (tea, a mocktail), or a food (such as pickles or a salad)—it's completely up to you. All the recipes in this chapter will be great inspiration for your inner mixologist. You can combine vinegar with any other ingredient, just avoid mixing it with sugar, honey, agave, or maple syrup, or fruit juice, because that would negate its effects. If you're making a drink and want to add some sweetness, you can add a few drops of stevia.

How to know if you're doing it right

Your vinegar hack should be **totally enjoyable and delicious**. If it burns your throat, or makes you uncomfortable in any way, you're not diluting the vinegar enough. Add more water, or reduce the quantity of vinegar to start with. (And if vinegar really isn't your thing, you can replace it with lemon—see page 106.)

Note: If you have stomach issues or your doctor recommends you don't do this hack, please do skip it. Just continue on with the savory breakfast this week.

Tips from the community

• The quality of a vinegar makes a big difference to how tasty it is. If you don't like the flavor of the vinegar you regularly use at home, try a different kind.

• Measuring your dosage of vinegar is also important, as it's common to make yourself a drink that is too strong if you just eyeball the quantity.

• The easiest time to take your daily vinegar is in the morning, with or before breakfast. You're more likely to remember it then.

• For those of you who would rather have your vinegar later in the day, the recipes for teas and mocktails help *a lot*. Try them. They are surprisingly tasty and easy.

• Sip on your vinegar while you're cooking a meal.

• The Hot Cinnamon Tea (page 130) is a community favorite! Try it!

• Make it a ritual, and try using a fancy glass!

Ask your body what it needs

Unsteady glucose levels are a common cause of cravings. Because of that, you may have spent years on a glucose roller coaster that has made you accustomed to needing a pastry at 10 a.m., coffee and sugar at 3 p.m., and ice cream after dinner. If you've always been on a glucose roller coaster (which most of us have), these urges will have become daily habits.

During this second week, things will change for the better, and I want you to pay close attention to how your body feels. As your glucose-dip-generated cravings dissipate, it's important to check in with your urges and question them.

At 10 a.m., pause and ask yourself if you really want that pastry or if, actually, you still feel full from breakfast and don't want the pastry anymore. At 3 p.m., check in with your energy levels—maybe you're no longer tired in the afternoons and can now skip your coffee and sugar. And so on. Don't take anything for granted! Get curious. Speak to your body. And listen. It's important to make sure you're eating what you want in the moment and not just out of habit. And if you do want the pastry, sugar, or ice cream, then by all means—enjoy it. Remember, in this Method, we don't restrict anything. Nothing is off-limits, nothing is bad. Just focus on the hacks and do what floats your boat the rest of the time. And if you want inspiration for full meals and desserts, you will find lots of my favorite recipes on pages 226–67.

Common questions from the community

When exactly should I have my vinegar? The bottom line is that *any time works*. As long as you're having one tablespoon a day, you're successfully completing this hack. You can have it in the morning when you're fasted, with or after your savory breakfast, during the day when you think of it, or before, during, or after lunch or dinner. *But* . . . if you happen to eat something starchy or sweet during the day, just know that having the vinegar ten minutes before that food will be extra powerful. If you forget to have it before, you can have it *while* you're eating or *after* the food, and it will still have a positive impact.

Can I take pills or gummies instead? If you want to try pills, be aware that you might need to swallow three or more to get the amount of acetic acid that is found in one tablespoon of vinegar (about 800mg). The chewable gummies that currently exist are definitely not a good move: they contain sugar (about 1g of sugar per gummy). So not only might they not work to flatten your glucose curves, they could actually lead to spikes. (I reached out to one leading apple cider vinegar gummy brand to ask for scientific backing for its claims—I didn't get an answer.) Maybe one day I'll make my own gummies that actually work.

Is there a limit to how much I can drink? Well, yes. A 29-year-old woman who consumed 16 tablespoons of vinegar every day for six years was admitted to the hospital because of very low levels of potassium, sodium, and bicarbonate. So don't do that. That's way too much. One tablespoon a day should be plenty!

Should I try to work up to having it before every meal? I'm not saying there is necessarily anything wrong with that, but you really don't need to. One tablespoon a day is a great objective that will give you benefits.

Which vinegar is best? All vinegars work: white, red, apple cider, balsamic, champagne, cherry, rice . . . The only ones to avoid are the very syrupy balsamic vinegars that are thick and aged. Those contain too much sugar to work.

Can I have pickles instead? Yes—you'll need a good handful of pickles. And if you go for store-bought, make sure they weren't pickled with sugar (check the ingredients on the label). I have lots of cool recipes showing you how to make your own on pages 124–29. At least with these you know what's gone into them, and they are ready immediately. They also keep in the fridge for up to four weeks.

Can I put vinegar on a salad instead of drinking it? Yes! I have delicious dressing recipes for you on pages 136–39.

How about kombucha? Kombucha has less than 1 percent acetic acid, which doesn't make it powerful enough to compete with regular vinegar (which is about 5 percent acetic acid). And if it's not homemade, it often has added sugar in it. That said, although it is not a spike slasher and therefore cannot be used *instead of* the regular vinegar, it still has some health benefits: it's a fermented food, so it contains beneficial bacteria that fuel the good microbes in our gut.

Can I have lime instead of lemon? Yes (for more on how to do this hack using citrus fruit, see the Lemon Option on page 106).

Can I have it with my stomach issues or heartburn? It depends—check with your doctor. And if there are any concerns, don't hesitate to either switch to the Lemon Option (page 106) or skip this hack entirely and continue with just the savory breakfast this week.

Can I have vinegar while pregnant or breastfeeding? Most standard vinegars are pasteurized and safe to consume during pregnancy or breastfeeding. However, apple cider vinegar is usually unpasteurized, which may present risks to pregnant women. Check with your doctor first.

I don't like the taste of vinegar. What should I do? Start with a small quantity, and work your way up. Or try white vinegar instead of apple cider vinegar (some people prefer it). Or try some of the mocktails and teas from the recipe section to come—they will probably surprise you. And if vinegar really doesn't work for you, try lemon juice instead (see page 106).

Why do the recipes recommend a straw? Even though diluted vinegar is not acidic enough to damage your teeth's enamel, I would suggest you drink it with a straw just to be safe. Never swig it straight from the bottle. As part of other foods, such as a vinaigrette, it's fine.

Are there any negative side effects to drinking one tablespoon of vinegar? You shouldn't experience any negative side effects as long as you stick to drinkable vinegar—i.e., vinegar with 5 percent acidity (cleaning vinegar has 6 percent acidity, so if it's next to the mops and toilet paper at the supermarket, don't drink it!).

Uh-oh, I forgot to drink vinegar before my meal. Is it too late? No! I do this all the time. No worries. You can still drink the vinegar during or after your meal.

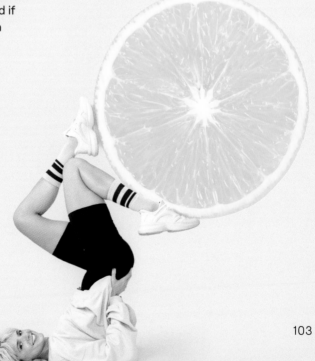

THE GG CLASSIC

What you need:

1 tablespoon apple cider vinegar or other vinegar you enjoy

A 2020 original. The most straightforward way to add vinegar to your day. Any time during the day works—but it's extra powerful if you have it before eating anything starchy or sweet. Some vinegars are less striking than others, so choose one that best suits your taste buds. Drink up, buttercup!

How to make it:

● Mix the **vinegar** and 1¼ cups/300ml of **water** in a tall glass. Ideally, drink the contents through a straw to protect your teeth's enamel. (If you find the taste too strong, start with 1 teaspoon instead of 1 tablespoon of vinegar.)

TIP: If you want, you can add a squeeze of lemon juice or ice cubes, or you can use sparkling water.

Serves: 1
GLUTEN-FREE, VEGAN

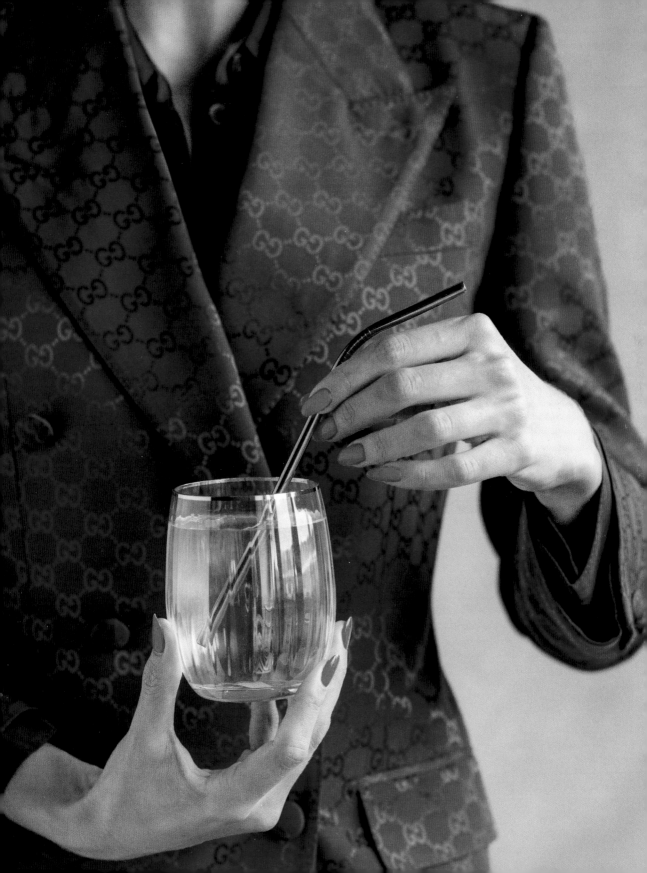

THE LEMON OPTION
(for those who can't stand vinegar)

What you need:

juice of ½ lemon

a few ice cubes (optional)

If vinegar is a no go (you just can't do it), then breeze through the vinegar hack by replacing it with lemon juice. Not as powerful on your glucose levels, but still helpful. You can also use lime juice instead of lemon.

How to make it:

● Mix the **lemon juice** with 1¼ cups/300ml of **water** in a tall glass, with some ice, too, if you like. You can use sparkling water instead, if you prefer. Ideally, drink the contents through a straw to protect your teeth's enamel. Alternatively, pour the contents of the glass into a water bottle (see The Emotional Support Water Bottle on page 112) and sip on it all day.

Serves: 1
GLUTEN-FREE, VEGAN

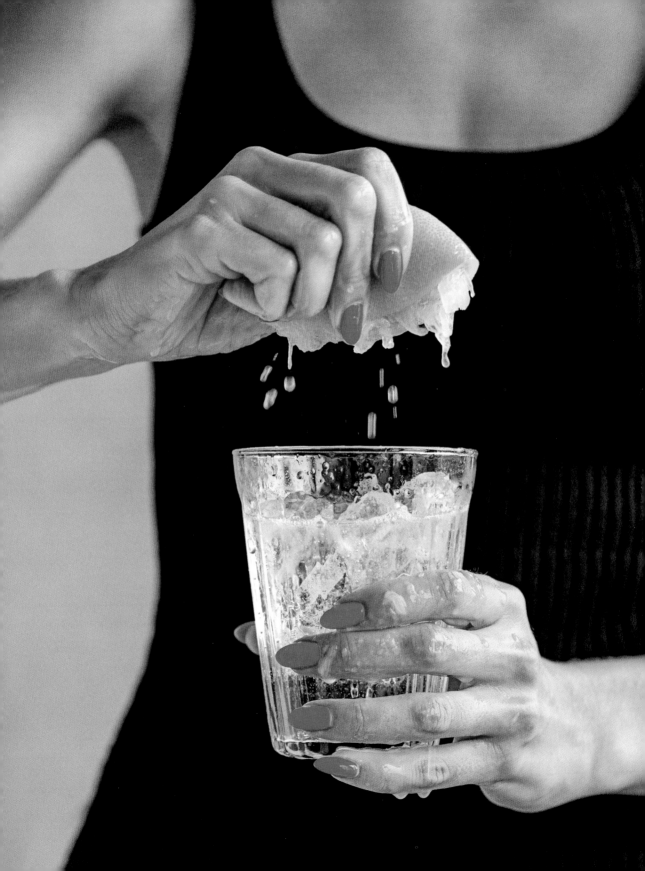

THE ICE-CUBE TRAY

What you need:

apple cider vinegar or other vinegar you enjoy

If you are someone who likes organizing things and doesn't want to dirty a spoon every day to measure out vinegar doses, this is for you: portion out your daily vinegar tablespoons into your ice-cube tray, and pop a cube into your drink of choice every day. Boom!

How to make it:

● Pour 1 tablespoon of **apple cider vinegar** into each hollow of an ice-cube tray and freeze. When frozen, add a cube to any drink you fancy—in a water bottle, glass, or mug!

Makes: as many as you have hollows in your ice-cube tray / Prep time: 5 min
GLUTEN-FREE, VEGAN

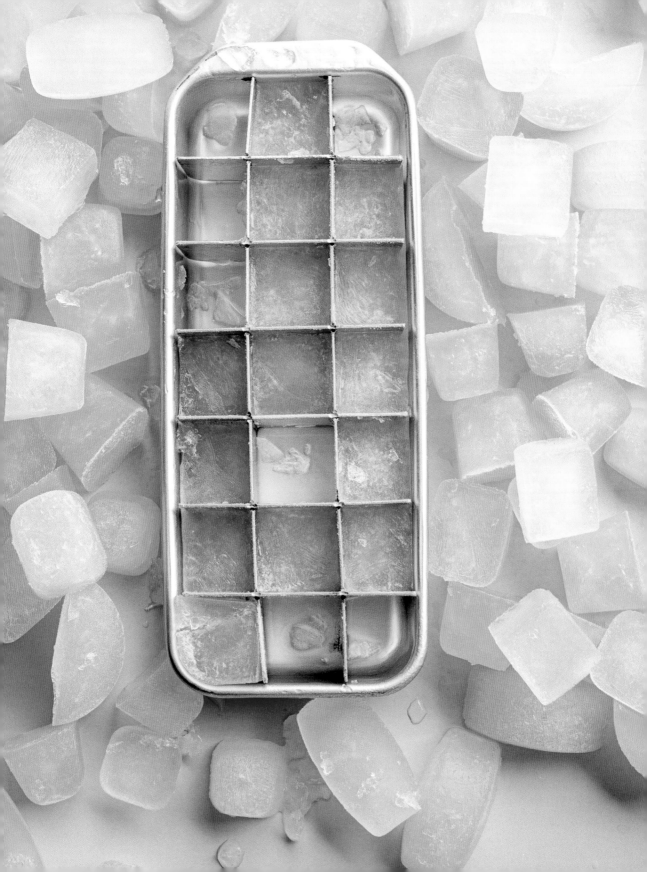

THE FLASK

What you need:

apple cider vinegar or other vinegar you enjoy

Or how to have your vinegar on the go.

How to make it:

● Pour several tablespoons of your favorite **vinegar** into your flask. Keep the flask in your bag and add 1 tablespoon of vinegar from the flask to any drink on the go—at the restaurant, the office, while traveling . . .

GLUTEN-FREE, VEGAN

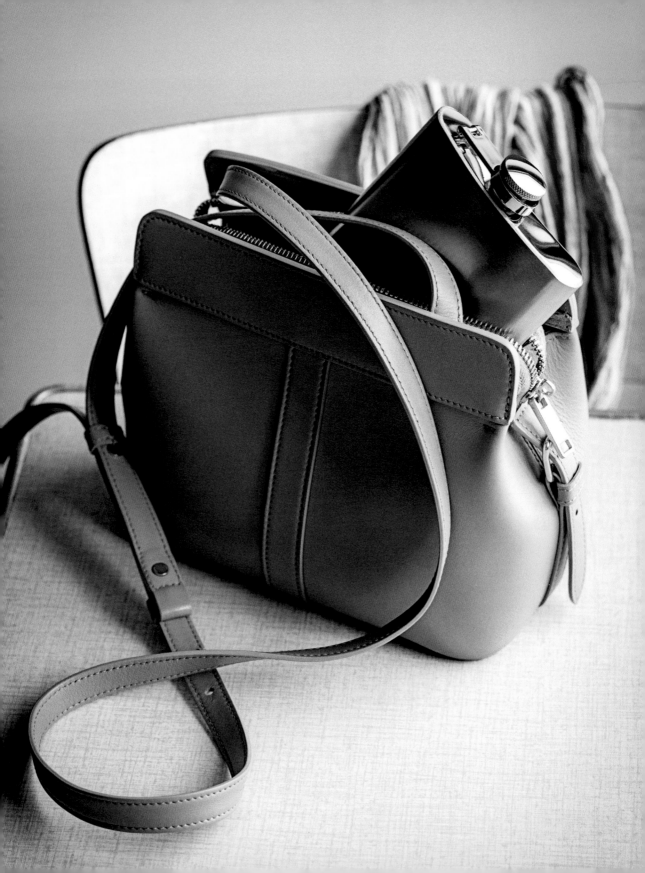

THE EMOTIONAL SUPPORT WATER BOTTLE

What you need:

1 tablespoon apple cider vinegar or other vinegar you enjoy

Here's another way to get your vinegar hack in: dilute a tablespoon in your water bottle, and sip on it throughout the day. Carry the water bottle with you like a teddy bear. Emotional support and glucose support combined.

How to make it:

● Mix the **vinegar** and 2¼ cups/500ml of **water** in your water bottle (or
use enough water to fill the bottle).

Serves: 1
GLUTEN-FREE, VEGAN

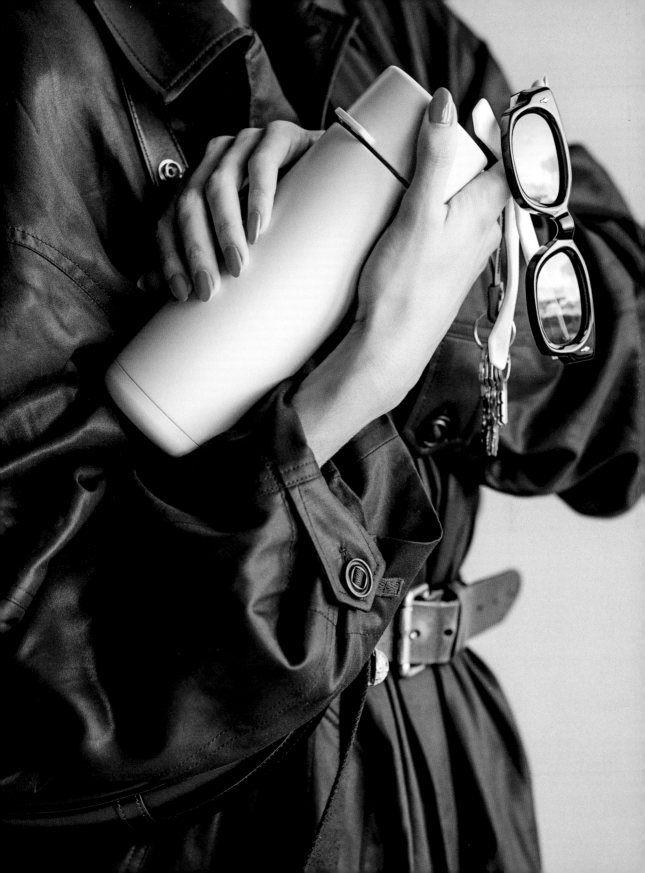

THE RESTAURANT VINEGAR DRINK

What you need:

a nice waiter/waitress

some vinegar

I'm often asked what you should do if you don't have vinegar with you and you want to complete your vinegar hack while at a restaurant. Good news: most restaurants have vinegar. Better news: you might get your whole party to pour some into their water glasses, too.

How to make it:

• Ask your waiter for **vinegar**—any kind—and pour 1 tablespoon into your glass of **water**. Drink it ideally before you start eating, but during the meal is also fine.

GLUTEN-FREE, VEGAN

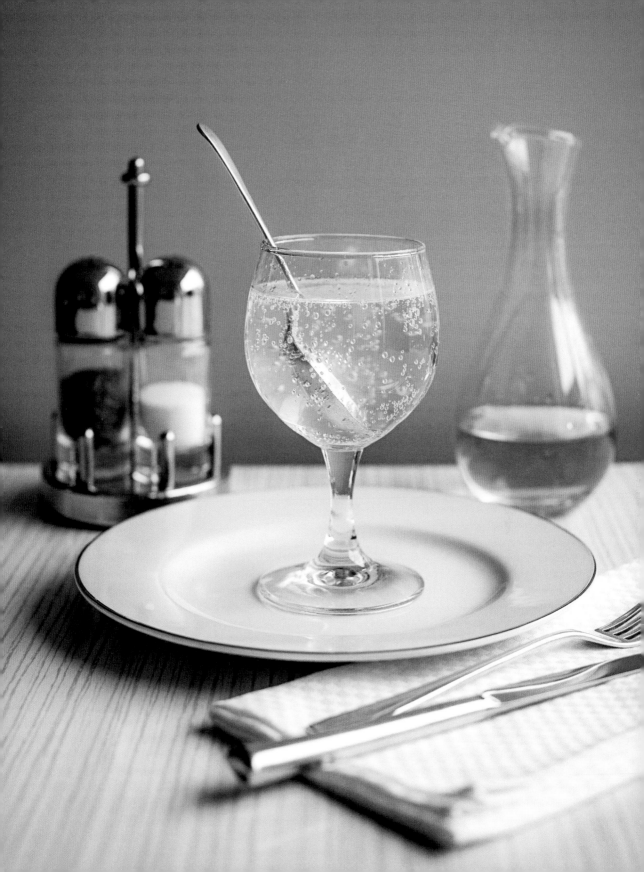

Try-me MOJITO SLUSHIE

What you need:

2 mint sprigs, stemmed, plus more for garnish

1 tablespoon apple cider vinegar

a handful of ice cubes
soda water, to top up

And so we begin a series of mocktails that check off your vinegar hack for the day, and make for a fun ritual. I know that you might be inclined to slide over these recipes, but give them a try. The participants in my pilot study told me that they made a big difference in helping them enjoy the vinegar hack.

How to make it:

● Blitz the **mint** leaves, **apple cider vinegar**, and **ice cubes** together in a blender until the mixture is like a slushy.

● Transfer the mixture to a cocktail glass, top up with **soda water**, garnish with mint leaves, and serve.

Serves: 1 / Prep time: 5 min
GLUTEN-FREE, VEGAN

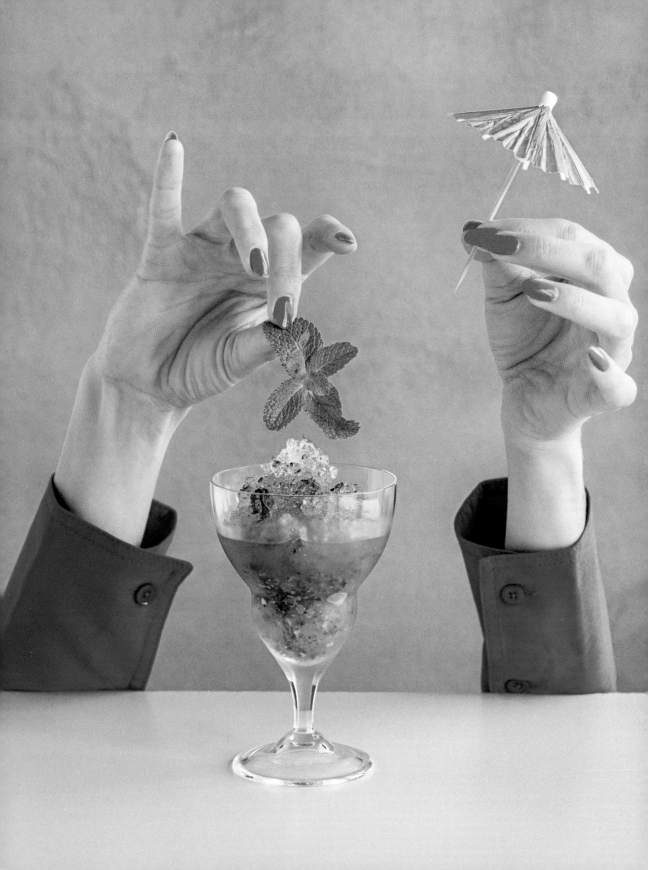

GINGER GIANT

What you need:

1¼-inch/3cm piece of ginger, peeled and finely grated

1 tablespoon apple cider vinegar

a few ice cubes
soda water, to top up

a slice of lime, for garnish (optional)

I love the concept of glucose hacks being gentle giants that we place throughout our day. They protect our glucose levels and free us up to do whatever we want. This particular giant leaves a tingle on the lips and heat in the throat. If you love ginger, start with two teaspoons of it, freshly grated. If you are new to it, start with one teaspoon and build up to two.

How to make it:

● Mix the grated **ginger** and **apple cider vinegar** together in a glass.

● Fill the glass with **ice cubes** and top up with **soda water**. A slice of lime makes a nice garnish, if you wish.

Serves: 1 / Prep time: 5 min
GLUTEN-FREE, VEGAN

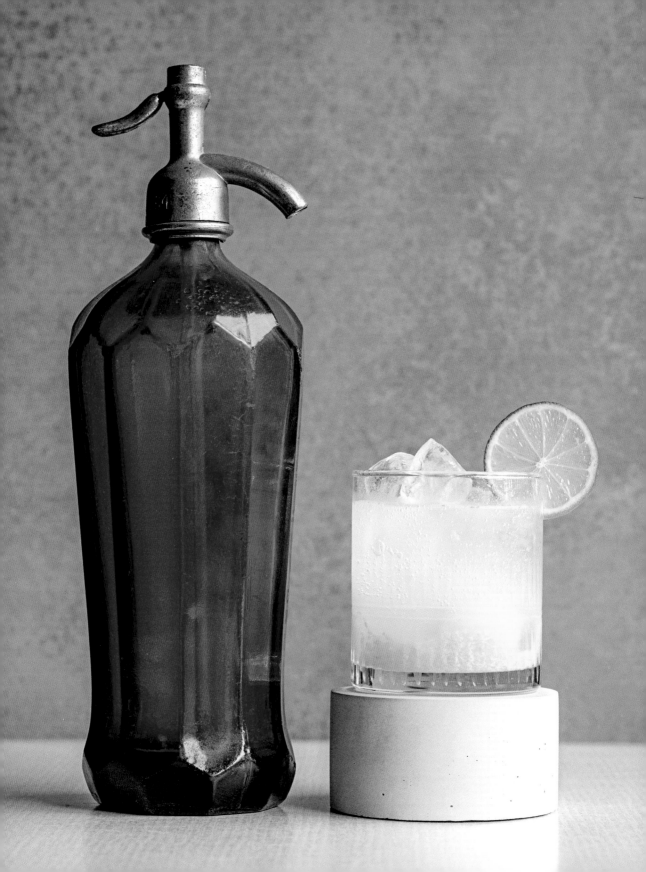

MOTHER APPLE SPRITZER

What you need:

1 teaspoon ground cinnamon

1 tablespoon apple cider vinegar

a few ice cubes
soda water, to top up

½ small apple, cored and sliced

All this talk of apple cider vinegar, but not enough credit to its birth mother: apples! Here they are, front and center. A super-tasty spritzer to sip, preferably while sitting under an apple tree. (If you do, send me a photo.)

How to make it:

● Mix the **cinnamon** and **apple cider vinegar** in a small bowl until fully combined (it takes a bit of mixing before the cinnamon completely blends in).

● Pour the mixture into a coupe glass. Add some **ice cubes** and some **soda water**. Finish with the slices of **apple**, and serve.

Makes: 1 portion / Prep time: 3 min
GLUTEN-FREE, VEGAN

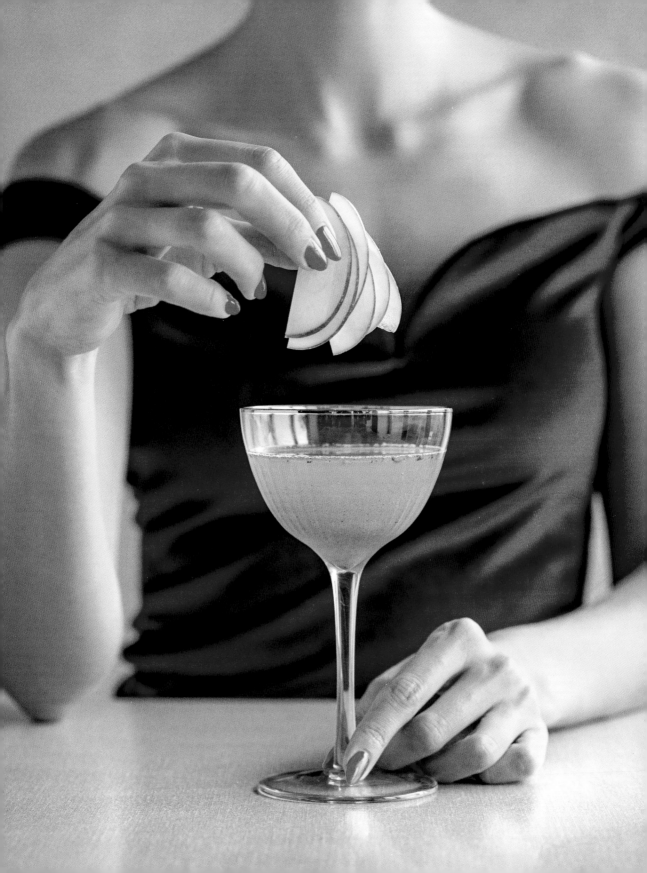

NOT-ORANGE-JUICE SPRITZER

What you need:

1-inch/2.5cm piece of ginger, peeled and roughly chopped

2 mint sprigs, stemmed, plus an optional extra sprig to garnish

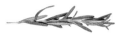

1 rosemary sprig, stemmed, plus an optional extra sprig to garnish

zest of 1 small unwaxed orange, plus an optional slice to garnish

¼ teaspoon ground turmeric

1 tablespoon apple cider vinegar

a few ice cubes

+ soda water, to top up

Looks like orange juice, is definitely not orange juice. Because orange juice (and all fruit juices for that matter) is a one-way ticket to a glucose roller coaster, whereas our friend here is a spike slasher.

How to make it:

● Place the **ginger**, **mint**, **rosemary**, **orange zest**, **turmeric**, and **apple cider vinegar** in a tall glass and use the end of a wooden spoon to gently mash everything together.

● Top up with **soda water**, then put some **ice cubes** in a fresh glass and strain the spritzer into it. Serve with a slice of orange and/or some mint or rosemary to garnish, if you wish.

Serves: 1 / Prep time: 5 min
GLUTEN-FREE, VEGAN

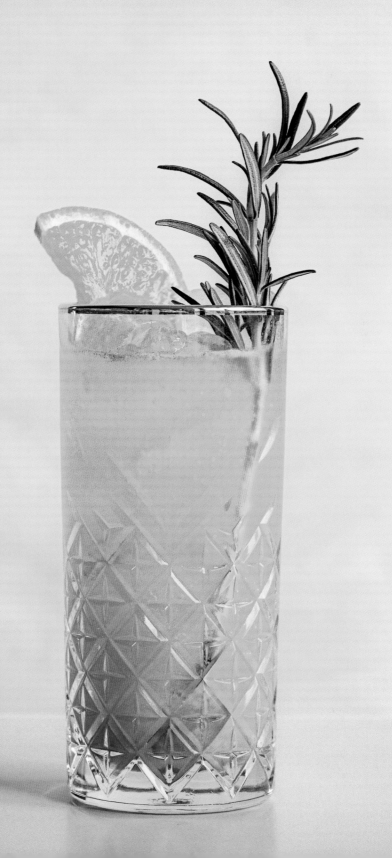

CUCUMBER *and* FENNEL PICKLES

What you need:

¾ cup plus 2 tablespoons/ 200ml apple cider vinegar

1 tablespoon fennel seeds

1 large cucumber, rinsed and thinly sliced

+ 1 tablespoon salt

Can we eat pickles to check off our vinegar hack? We sure can. The best way to ensure they will steady our glucose is to make them ourselves (store-bought pickles sometimes have sugar in them). All the pickle recipes on the next pages will be ready for immediate consumption. Eating about five pickles will give you your one-tablespoon daily vinegar goal.

How to make it:

● Pour the **apple cider vinegar** into a saucepan. Add the **fennel seeds**, ¼ cup/60ml of **water**, and the **salt** and place the pan on medium heat. Bring the mixture to a boil, then immediately remove the pan from the heat and set it aside for the liquid to cool slightly.

● Meanwhile, pack the sliced **cucumber** into a sterilized 1–pint/500ml jar (see note). Pour the cooled liquid from the saucepan (including the seeds) into the jar to cover the cucumber slices, seal the jar, and refrigerate. The pickles are ready to use immediately, although the flavor will intensify over time. Use the pickles within 4 weeks.

A note on sterilizing jars: Preheat the oven to 275°F. Wash the jars and lids with clean, soapy water and rinse (but don't dry) them. Place the jars and lids upside down on a baking sheet and transfer them to the oven for 15–20 minutes. Fill and seal the jars while they are still hot.

Makes: 1 x 1-pint/500ml jar / Prep time: 15 min
GLUTEN-FREE, VEGAN

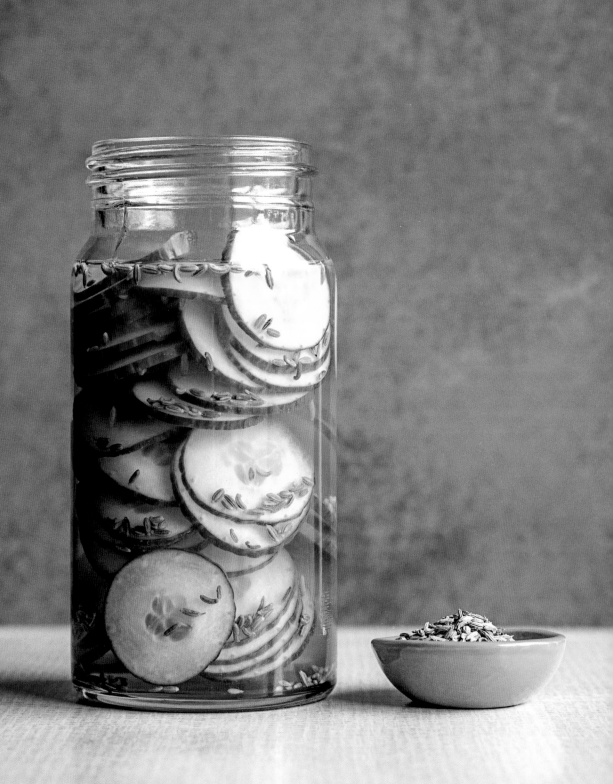

CAULIFLOWER *and* ZA'ATAR PICKLES

What you need:

¾ cup plus 2 tablespoons/ 200ml apple cider vinegar

1½ tablespoons za'atar

1 small cauliflower, stalks discarded, broken into small florets

+ 1 tablespoon salt

This one is a beauty. Eating five cauliflower florets will count as your daily one-tablespoon goal. Easy to nibble on while cooking a meal, or to add to your dinner plate as your protective friend.

How to make it:

● Pour the **apple cider vinegar** into a small saucepan. Add the **za'atar** and **salt** and place the pan on medium heat. Bring the liquid to a boil, then immediately remove the pan from the heat.

● Pack the **cauliflower** florets into a sterilized 1-pint/500ml jar (see note on page 124) and pour in the boiling liquid to completely cover the florets (the boiling liquid will soften and slightly cook the cauliflower). Seal the jar with the lid and let the pickling liquid cool. You can eat the pickles immediately, although they will benefit from 1 hour in the pickling liquid first, and will get stronger over time. Use within 4 weeks.

Makes: 1 x 1-pint/500ml jar / Prep time: 15 min
GLUTEN-FREE, VEGAN

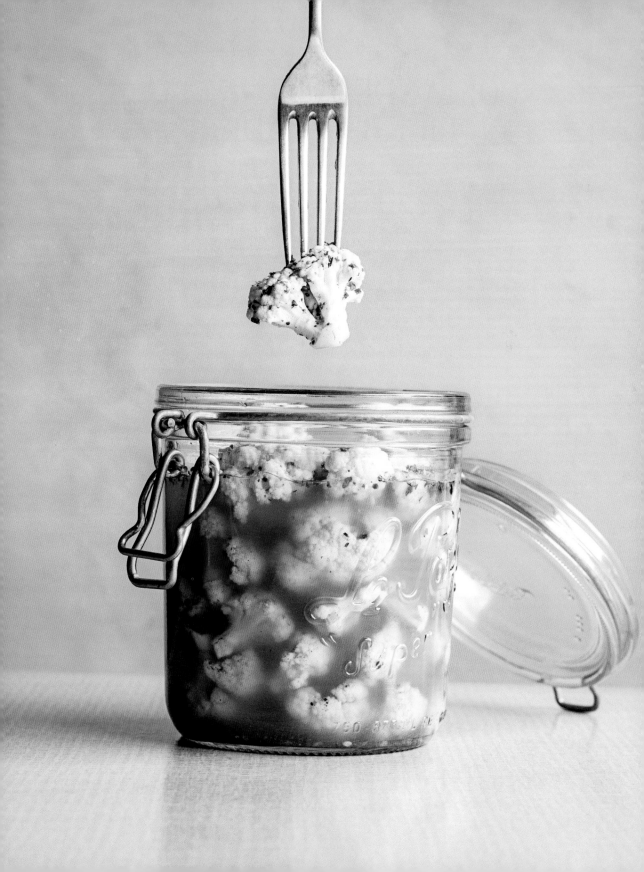

CORIANDER *and* ORANGE PICKLED RADISH

What you need:

¾ cup plus 2 tablespoons/ 200ml apple cider vinegar

4 strips of unwaxed orange peel

1 tablespoon coriander seeds

7 ounces/200g radishes, thinly sliced

+ 1 tablespoon salt

In my opinion, the most impressive jar of pickles to have in your fridge. And a perfect companion to the Today I'm Fancy Salmon Toast (page 64). If you want to knock out your breakfast and vinegar hacks in one, add five radish slices to that toast or any other breakfast recipe.

How to make it:

● Pour the **apple cider vinegar** into a small saucepan. Add the **orange peel**, **coriander seeds**, and **salt** and place the pan on medium heat. Bring the liquid to a boil, then immediately remove the pan from the heat. Set it aside and let the liquid cool slightly.

● Pack the **radish** slices into a sterilized 1-pint/500ml jar, pour in the cooled liquid (including the seeds and peel) to cover, then seal and refrigerate. You can eat the pickles immediately, although they will benefit from 1 hour in the pickling liquid first, and will get stronger over time. Use within 4 weeks.

Makes: 1 x 1-pint/500ml jar / Prep time: 15 min
GLUTEN-FREE, VEGAN

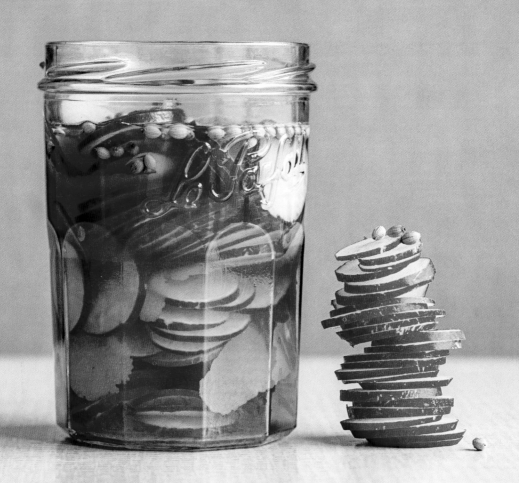

THE HOT CINNAMON TEA

What you need:

1 teaspoon apple cider vinegar

½ teaspoon ground cinnamon
hot water (almost boiling)
cinnamon stick, to garnish (optional)

Can you have vinegar in teas? Yes, you can! And if you're a little shy about this whole vinegar thing, this community-favorite warming recipe is a lovely place to start. The cinnamon and hot water complement the vinegar beautifully.

How to make it:

● In a mug, mix the **apple cider vinegar** and **cinnamon** together so that they are well combined. Pour in the **hot water**, stir, then garnish with a cinnamon stick, if you wish. Enjoy!

Serves: 1 / Prep time: 5 min
GLUTEN-FREE, VEGAN

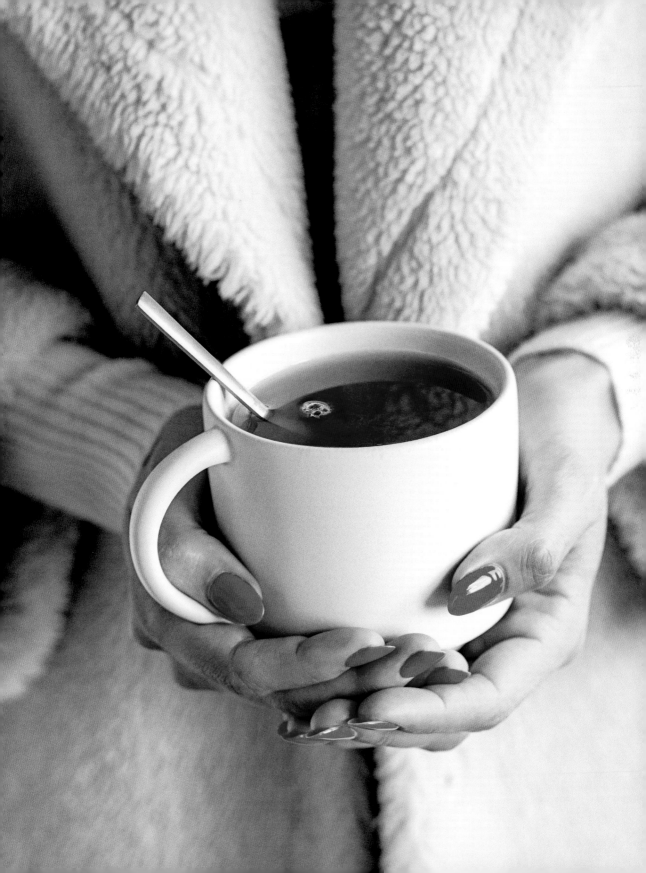

TURMERIC AND PEPPER TEA

What you need:

1 tablespoon apple cider vinegar

¼ teaspoon ground turmeric

½ teaspoon ground black pepper
hot water (almost boiling)

Well, good morning to you, too! When waking up is hard to do, may I suggest reaching for a cup of Turmeric and Pepper Tea? It's like a splash of cold water on the face, but vastly more enjoyable.

How to make it:

● In a mug, mix the **apple cider vinegar**, **turmeric**, and **black pepper** together and top up the mug with the **hot water**.

Serves: 1 / Prep time: 5 min
GLUTEN-FREE, VEGAN

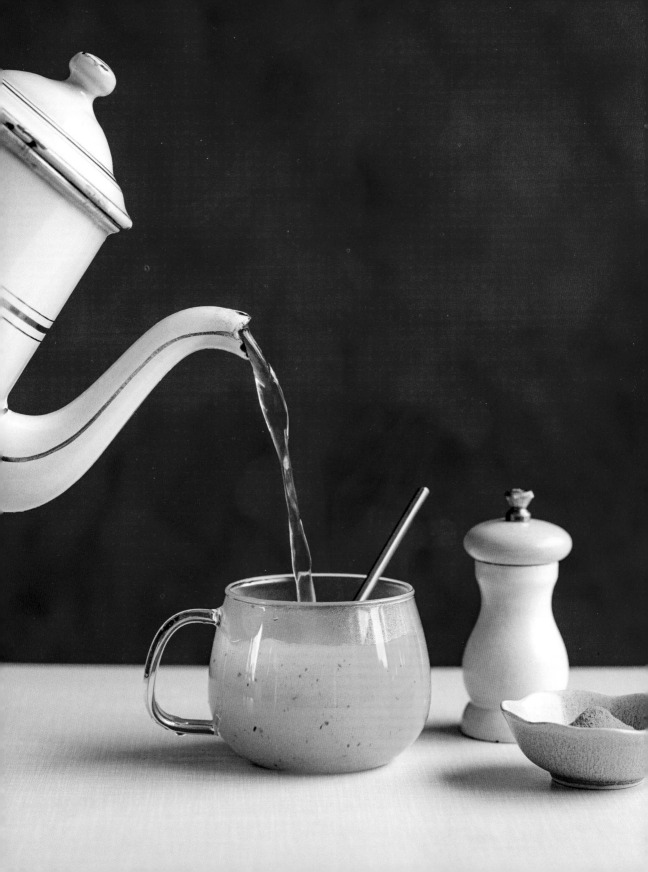

Next-level FIRE CIDER

What you need:

2-inch/5cm piece of ginger, peeled and roughly chopped

1 red or green chile, halved lengthwise

½ unwaxed orange, thinly sliced, then each slice quartered

1 teaspoon ground turmeric

½ teaspoon cayenne pepper

¾ cup plus 2 tablespoons/ 200ml apple cider vinegar

Are you the kind of person who likes a challenge? Then jump into the ring and try this little fiery beauty. Add one tablespoon of this hot and spicy Fire Cider to some soda water for a cool drink, or to a mug of hot water for a tea; or combine it with a few tablespoons of olive oil and mustard for a mind-blowing salad dressing. Note: You need to make this recipe two days in advance so the ingredients have time to meld and spark.

How to make it:

● Place **all of the ingredients** into a sterilized 1-pint/500ml jar (see note on page 124). Seal the jar with a lid, then shake well and refrigerate. The "cider" is ready to use after 2–3 days and will keep for up to 4 weeks. Shake well before using.

Makes: 1 x 1-pint/500ml jar / Prep time: 10 min
GLUTEN-FREE, VEGAN

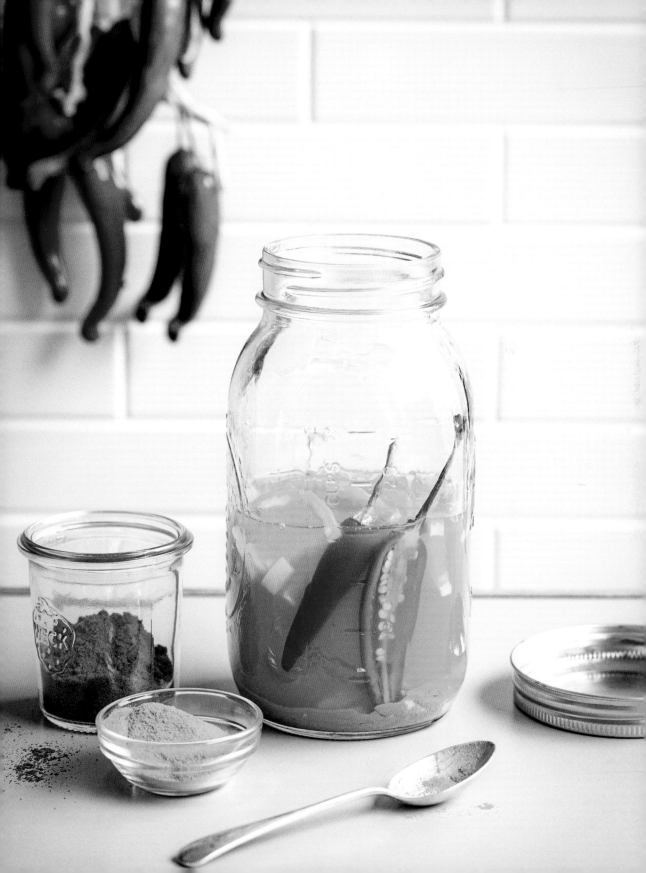

OREGANO DRESSING

What you need:

2 tablespoons
apple cider
vinegar

2 tablespoons
Dijon mustard

1 tablespoon
dried oregano

+ 6 tablespoons/90ml olive oil
+ salt and pepper

Another easy way to get your vinegar hack in is by having it as a dressing on your food. The next few pages showcase my favorite ways to dress up my dishes and reduce their glucose spike.

How to make it:

● Place the **the apple cider vinegar**, **Dijon mustard**, **oregano**, and **olive oil** in a small jar, season well with **salt** and **pepper**, then seal the jar. Shake everything up until it's all emulsified. Refrigerate until needed.

Makes: 2 servings / Prep time: 5 min
GLUTEN-FREE, VEGAN

PERFECT PARMESAN DRESSING

What you need:

2 tablespoons
apple cider
vinegar

¼ cup/30g finely grated
Parmesan

12 basil leaves,
roughly torn

+ 6 tablespoons/90ml
olive oil
+ salt and pepper

Listen team, it's not my fault, I was raised on Parmesan. I calculated that I've probably eaten 330 pounds of it so far in my 30 years of existence. That's about the weight of a panda bear. So you will see it in this book *a lot*. Apologies in advance. Good news is, it makes for a mean vinegar dressing.

How to make it:

● Place the **apple cider vinegar**, grated **Parmesan**, **basil leaves**, and **olive oil** in a small bowl and season with **salt** and **pepper**. Use an immersion blender to blitz the mixture until it is smooth and beautifully green. The dressing is best used immediately, but it will keep in the fridge for 2–3 days, although it may lose some of its vibrant green color in that time.

Makes: 2 servings / Prep time: 7 min
GLUTEN-FREE, VEGETARIAN

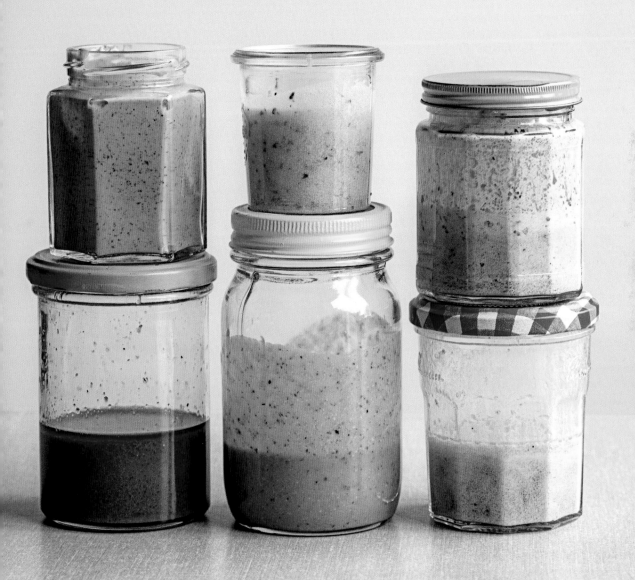

HOT SRIRACHA DRESSING

What you need:

2 tablespoons sesame oil

2 tablespoons apple cider vinegar

2 tablespoons sriracha

2 tablespoons soy sauce (or tamari, if you're gluten-free)

4 teaspoons English mustard

+ pepper to taste

Some like it hot, some like it cold, some like it in the pot seven days old. Some also like to use nursery rhymes to snag your attention. If you fall into the some-like-it-hot category, this vinegar dressing is for you. Try it on a colorful coleslaw, with roasted red peppers, or on some arugula and walnuts for a fresh salad that completes your vinegar hack for the day.

How to make it:

● Place **all of the ingredients** in a jar. Place a lid on the jar to seal, then shake the dressing until it's emulsified. Refrigerate until needed (you may need to give it an extra shake before using).

Makes: 2 servings / Prep time: 5 min
GLUTEN-FREE (if using tamari), VEGAN

HARISSA *and* YOGURT DRESSING

What you need:

2 tablespoons full-fat Greek yogurt

1 tablespoon harissa paste

2 tablespoons apple cider vinegar

+ 1 tablespoon olive oil
+ salt and pepper to taste

I told you that vinegar would be way easier and more fun than you thought. Please meet this gorgeous dressing. I'm a sucker for yogurt dressings on some fresh kale, or with roasted veggies.

How to make it:

● Place **all of the ingredients** in a jar, then seal the jar with a lid. Shake the jar until the contents are thoroughly combined. Refrigerate, and use the dressing within 5 days.

Makes: 2 servings / Prep time: 5 min
GLUTEN-FREE, VEGETARIAN

OLIVE *and* CAPER DRESSING

What you need:

2 tablespoons apple cider vinegar

1 teaspoon capers, drained

3 pitted green olives

2 teaspoons Dijon mustard

+ 3 tablespoons olive oil
+ salt and pepper to taste

Not all heroes wear capes. Some wear capers. This dressing is a bit of a curve ball, but if it pleases your taste buds you might be making it every day. It's a great one to try when you are feeling adventurous.

How to make it:

● Place **all of the ingredients** in a bowl and mash them together with a fork until emulsified (or you can finely chop the **capers** and **olives** and mix them like that). Refrigerate until needed.

Makes: 2 servings / Prep time: 7 min
GLUTEN-FREE, VEGAN

GREEN GODDESS DRESSING-DIP

What you need:

½ small ripe avocado, pitted

a small bunch of cilantro

juice of ½ lime

 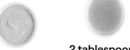

1 tablespoon Dijon mustard

2 tablespoons apple cider vinegar

+ 2 tablespoons olive oil
+ salt and pepper to taste

Goddesses work together. Prepare this as a dip for raw veggies or to top off a bowl full of greens. Or if you like it as much as I do, eat it with a spoon. Vinegar? Check. Deliciousness? Check. A silky smooth, almost scoopable dressing.

How to make it:

● Place **all of the ingredients** into a food processor and blitz until smooth. The dressing is best used right away but will keep for 24 hours, covered, in the fridge (it may discolor, but will taste the same in that time).

Makes: 2 servings / Prep time: 5 min
GLUTEN-FREE, VEGAN

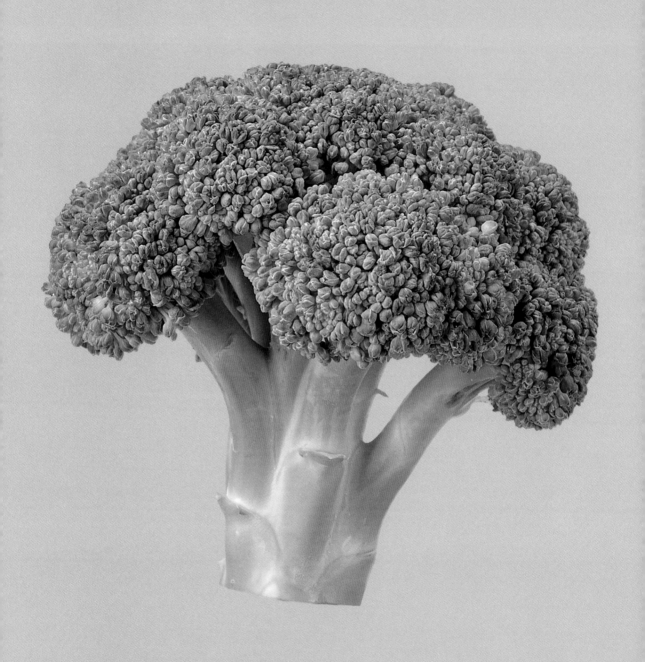

VEGGIE STARTER

Fabulous things come to those
who start Week 3 . . . it's time to meet
a glucose superwoman: fiber!

TESTIMONIALS FROM THE COMMUNITY

"Feeling less bloated and sleeping better. I've learned a lot throughout these first three weeks, about food, my body, and some reactions and responses that I didn't understand until now. One thing I never did was eat veggies first, and it makes a big difference to my appetite."

"I'll be 65 in January, and this is how I'm going to probably be eating the rest of my life!"

"I feel better and better every day. The unwanted facial hair on my chin has reduced."

"My awareness of how what I eat affects the way my body feels has dramatically increased. For example, I skipped the veggie starter and vinegar for one meal, and I almost went into a 'food coma'— meaning I didn't eat more, but the meal got me super sleepy, drained, and cranky. Mind-boggling realization for me!"

"I'm so grateful for this Method. My quality of life and overall health have been improving since Week 1."

"The veggie starter has become a must-have for me and I feel so much better."

"I noticed I had fewer nighttime cravings when I had a veggie starter before dinner."

"After this week, I can't start a meal without a veggie starter . . . it just doesn't make sense not to prepare my body for the food I will eat."

"I didn't see much of a change during vinegar week, but now my cravings are reduced significantly. Veggie starters are a nonnegotiable. I love the program and how easy the hacks are. They are now a habit, and that is the key to why it's so successful!"

"My waistline has reduced and I feel lighter and happier. I am able to eat without guilt and absolutely enjoy the veggie starters."

"So now my kids eat savory breakfast, and they eat veggie starters: great habits to make at an early stage in life."

"I thought this week was going to be challenging, but it turned out great and we are being creative with it."

"I'm so thrilled that I've learned how to handle the 4 p.m. munchies. Now I just grab a veggie starter and consider it predinner instead of feeling like I'm 'ruining my dinner' with other snacks."

"I now have stable energy levels throughout the day (I felt so tired every day after breakfast and in the afternoon or after some meals, and never knew why or how to fix that, but now I do). I can finally go longer between meals without getting dizzy, hangry, or having cravings (this is the biggest change for me, because I often suffered from dizziness and felt shaky when I was hungry, which I hated because I knew I had to get food as soon as possible and didn't know how to change that cycle)."

"Adding in a veggie starter rather than bread/chips before meals (even if I'm just grabbing some celery while cooking) made the biggest difference to how I felt after the total mealtime—no crash or dizziness an hour later."

"Eating my veggies first is reducing anxiety about what I must or must not eat. With the veggie starter I know I'm helping myself. I think just about that."

"I feel a definite improvement overall in mood and brain fog."

"One amazing difference was that recently I went to catch up with a friend and we had a couple of glasses of wine. Over the past year, I was finding that even one glass would impact my sleep so I was almost completely avoiding it— and while I know it's not a health drink anyway, it was to the point where I just felt I couldn't enjoy a glass once in a while. The other night, I had a veggie starter and a strong lemon water before going out. We ordered olives and cheese with the wine. I managed to enjoy the evening and, even better, was still able to sleep relatively well that night! Amazing!"

"It's so much easier eating veggies before a meal than I thought. I just keep them ready-cut in my fridge. I definitely have more energy."

Your objective for Week 3

Congratulations for making it halfway through our adventure together! At this point, your glucose is stabilizing, inflammation is reducing, and aging is slowing down. Your body is experiencing a profound positive change from the inside. You're helping your brain feel better today and helping your body ward off disease long term. You can be very proud.

This week's hack? Adding fiber to the beginning of our meals. A true goddess for our glucose curves, fiber is found mostly in vegetables. So here's the plan: **for the next two weeks, before one of your meals during the day, you will add a plate of veggies to the *start* of your meal.** This means *adding* food to your usual meals. I call it "a veggie starter." This veggie starter should make up about 30 percent of your meal.

It doesn't matter if the veggies are cooked, raw, dressed, or plain. You don't need to wait between your veggie starter and the rest of your meal, and you don't need to change the rest of your meal at all. You can even combine your veggie starter with a vinegar-based dressing, to check off two hacks in one. I've noted which recipes combine both (for example, the recipes on pages 152 and 168).

During the pilot experiment, many participants reported to me—to their surprise—that this hack was one of the hardest to do, because of the amount of preparation needed. So over the following pages, I have included lots of my favorite recipes for inspiration. They are all super simple to prepare. Indeed, many of them are quick assembly jobs: no cooking required. I recommend you plan for the next two weeks of veggie starters and make a detailed shopping list. You might be surprised how many veggies you actually need! And remember—we are also continuing with our savory breakfast and our vinegar hack from Weeks 1 and 2.

The science

Fiber is a plant-made substance found abundantly in vegetables. While it is helpful to incorporate fiber in our diet at any time, when eaten at the *beginning* of a meal, it has a particularly powerful impact on our glucose levels.

As we saw earlier, when fiber arrives in our upper intestine before other foods, it performs an amazing transformation: it deploys itself against the walls of our intestine, forming a viscous, protective mesh that stays in place for a few hours. This mesh then reduces the absorption of any glucose molecules that make their way into our digestive system during the rest of the meal: in this way it reduces the speed and velocity at which glucose arrives into our bloodstream, and reduces the glucose spike of the meal.

After your veggie starter, you can eat anything you usually eat, knowing that because the protective fiber mesh is there, there will be less of a glucose spike from your meal. To give you an idea, a study that simply flipped the order in which the foods were eaten during a meal showed that by putting the veggies first (and the carbs last), **the glucose spike of the meal was decreased by up to 75 percent**. This was achieved without changing *what* was in the meal at all, just by placing the veggies first and harnessing the power of the fiber they contain. Remarkable.

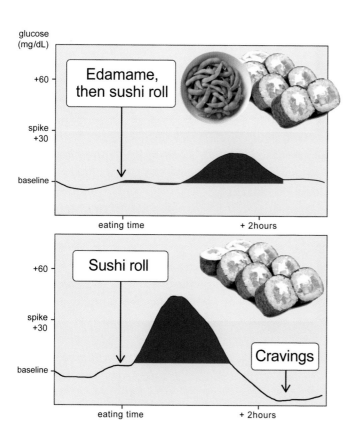

The powerful effect of a veggie starter on the glucose spike of a meal

How to make your own veggie starter

Veggie starters can be as simple (10 to 12 olives) or as fancy (for example, Baked Fennel, see page 192) as you want. I have more than 30 recipe ideas to inspire you.

If you'd like to make your own, here's what to do: pick your favorite veggie; prepare it your favorite way (raw, cooked, baked . . .); dress it with some proteins or fats, if you want (although avoid adding sugar to it); and eat it before the meal of your choice.

If you're eating at a restaurant, ask for a side salad at the beginning of your meal, or pick a starter that is vegetable-based, or look at the "sides" section of the menu: there is usually a veggie side that you can ask for and eat first: sautéed spinach or coleslaw or green beans . . .

If you are traveling, bring with you a bag of baby carrots, or some cherry tomatoes or cucumber slices in a zip-top bag. Ta-da!

How to know if you're doing it right

You'll know you're doing this hack properly if the veggie starter makes up **about 30 percent of your overall food quantity for that meal**. Depending on the size of your meals, you can adjust the recipe portions to hit this goal. If you have some starter left over, for example, save it for the next day. Your veggie starters may take a little bit of prep—but making batches and keeping some raw veggies in your fridge for when you are on the go will help.

Then, as you eat your veggies, picture the fiber from them arriving in your digestive system and setting up camp there to protect you for the rest of the meal. You might find that you eat less of your regular meal afterward; **however, eating less afterward is not the objective.** I encourage you to eat just as you normally do and to just add this veggie starter to the front end of your meal.

If your meal already contains veggies, you can turn them into a veggie starter simply by eating those veggies first, before you tuck into anything else on your plate.

Tips from the community

- Do as much prep as you can in advance. Make big batches of veggies, and keep them in the fridge for the whole week.

- Pick the meal in your day that is most convenient for you to add your veggie starter to. In the community, people are split on this almost equally: about 50 percent have their veggie starter before their lunch, and about 50 percent before their dinner. A handful of people have it before breakfast.

- Adding vinegar to your veggie starter dressing is a really easy way to get your vinegar hack done if you struggle with having that separately.

- The baby radish veggie starter (page 184) is hailed as a family favorite—for kids and parents alike.

- If you're not used to eating vegetables, you might experience some bloating as your gut gets used to the new fiber. If that's the case, choose cooked vegetables instead of raw veggies to begin with, as they may be easier on your system.

- There is no need to embrace a new variety of veggies with this hack. Any veggies work, so if it's easier for you, just pick your routine favorite way of having veggies, and enjoy that every day.

- As long as you have had your veggie starter, you can also have extra veggies during the rest of the meal.

- Veggie starters are easy to share: put raw veggies on the table for your whole family, or distribute them to your kids to munch on as you are preparing a meal.

Common questions from the community

What comes first, vinegar drink or veggie starter? If you are completing your vinegar hack and veggie starter hack at the same meal, then ideally have your vinegar drink first, veggie starter second. Or you can combine both by adding a vinegar-based dressing to your veggie starter.

How many veggies should I eat? Try to have your veggie starter make up about 30 percent of your overall meal volume. That's the goal. If one day you don't have time and you can only have a couple of cherry tomatoes, that's okay—a little bit of veggie starter is still better than none at all.

Can I do veggie starters at breakfast time? Absolutely! This week asks you to add a veggie starter to one of your meals per day, and it can absolutely be breakfast—although, most people are not very excited about having veggies first thing in the morning, so lunch and dinner are more popular choices.

How long should I wait between my veggie starter and my main meal? You don't have to wait at all, but if you do want to wait, up to 90 minutes is about the upper limit. Which means that if you want to have your veggie starter at home and then go out for dinner, you can do that!

I forgot to do my veggie starter today; what should I do? It's not a problem—it happens to all of us. There are a lot of things to remember to do, so it's normal if things slip your mind. Just continue tomorrow. Remember—as long as you use the hacks 80 percent of the time, the Method will work. Do also use the workbook on pages 27–35 to help you keep track of how you are doing.

Does sauerkraut count as a veggie starter? Yes—sauerkraut is made from cabbage, and cabbage is a (delicious) vegetable.

Do pickles count? Yes, pickles are veggies, and you can have them as a veggie starter. Make sure to increase your portion so they are about 30 percent of your meal's size. And some more good news: pickles also count as your vinegar hack! Just make sure, if your pickles are store-bought, that they don't contain sugar. To make your own, see pages 124–29.

Do olives, avocados, lentils, and legumes count? Yes. For the olives, have 10 to 12 of them—in a pinch, they do the job.

Can it be soup? Chunky soup works (see page 194 for my 5-Min Soup recipe). A highly blended soup isn't the best because in the blending process, fiber particles are pulverized, rendering them less effective at creating the protective mesh.

Can my veggies be pureed? Ideally not because pureeing also hurts the fiber particles. But you may not want to use your teeth (or maybe you just came back from the dentist), in which case, see No-Teeth Bean Puree on page 176.

I ate my veggie starter and now I'm not hungry anymore for the rest of my meal. Is that okay? Yes, that is fine, and it happens! I'd recommend reducing the portion size of your veggie starter in the future so that you still have room for the rest of your meal. But it's totally okay.

How many times a day should I have a veggie starter? Once a day is your objective. But if you can do it for both lunch and dinner and you want to, that will help your glucose even more.

How do I combine vinegar with my veggie starter? Simple: pick your favorite vinegar, and add one tablespoon of it to your veggie starter. You can also add one of last week's vinegar dressings (pages 136–39).

Can my veggie starter have dressing or extra ingredients on it? Yes, it will make it tastier. Olive oil, yogurt, vinegar, mustard, herbs, and spices are all great. You can also add anything that is protein and fat (cheese, nuts, meats, fish). As long as you're not adding mountains of it (one cherry tomato covered in a pound of cheese doesn't really count as a veggie starter), and as long as what you're adding doesn't contain anything sweet or starchy, you're good to go!

Should I eat all my veggies first, then all the proteins, then all the carbs? No, you don't need to do that—even though that is the scientifically proven ideal way to eat the elements of a meal for our glucose (see the first hack in my previous book, *Glucose Revolution*). But in the context of this Method, we are focusing only on veggies first. The rest of your meal you can eat in whatever order you like: all mixed together, or however you want, and you can add more veggies in, too.

Won't adding calories to a meal with this starter make me gain weight? Any extra calories from a veggie starter are good calories to add. They will keep you satiated, reduce cravings, reduce insulin release, and reduce inflammation. These are positive changes that improve our health and can lead to weight loss.

Can my meal be just the veggie starter? If you feel like it, it's no problem. You may want to add a serving of protein to have after the starter. Also check out our main dish recipes for inspiration (pages 226–51).

What should I eat as a main meal after my veggie starter? Anything!

Why dessert is a good idea

In Week 1, we learned about savory breakfasts and how avoiding eating sugar in the morning is the key to steadying our glucose. This week, we are learning that it's best to start a meal with vegetables to reduce the spike of starches and sugars coming afterward. These two hacks are teaching us an important lesson: things that contain glucose—starches and sugars—should not be the first things in our mouth when we are fasted or sitting down to eat.

The best time to eat sweet foods is *after* a meal, as dessert. When sugar comes last, at the end of a meal, the other foods already in our system blunt the glucose spike that the sugar creates. And if the meal started with veggies, that's even better: the protective fiber mesh will play a big role in slowing down the absorption of whatever sugar is to come.

So if you want to eat a cookie or your favorite chocolate ice cream, try not to eat it on an empty stomach; *eat it as dessert*. This means you'll be able to enjoy it with less risk of a cravings roller coaster—a very powerful place to be.

EXPRESS FIBER

What you need:

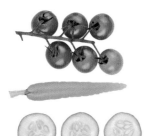

5 cherry tomatoes, 5 baby carrots, or 5 cucumber slices (or a combination of all three)

3 heaping tablespoons hummus (optional)

No time, no energy, no problem! Snag a few veggies from your fridge, pair them with a yummy dip (or not!), and there you have it: a super-quick, super-helpful veggie starter. Ideally, your veggie starter makes up about one-third of your meal, but when that's not possible, even a few cherry tomatoes out of the fridge will count, and are better than not having any at all.

How to make it:

● Assemble the **tomatoes, carrots, or cucumber** (or any other veggie). Add some hummus to a dipping bowl if you want (or use any other dip you fancy).

● Pop them in your mouth.

Makes: 1 portion / Prep time: 3 min
GLUTEN-FREE, VEGAN

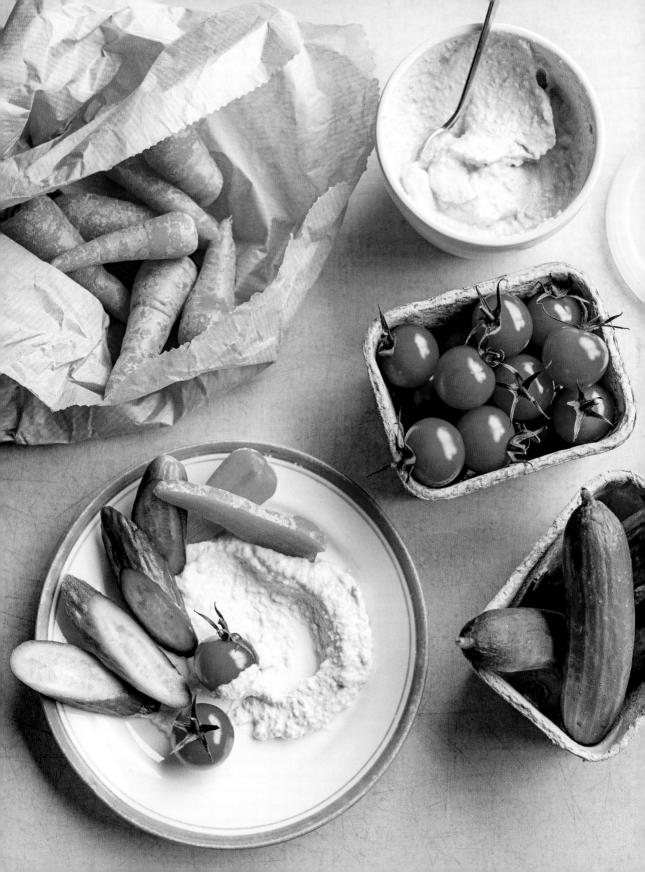

CAULIFLOWER SALAD

COUNTS AS YOUR VINEGAR HACK FOR THE DAY AS WELL

What you need:

½ small cauliflower, roughly chopped (use the leaves, too)

2 teaspoons Dijon mustard

1 tablespoon apple cider vinegar

¾ ounce/20g Cheddar, crumbled or cut into cubes

a handful of flat-leaf parsley, stems trimmed, leaves roughly chopped

+ 4 tablespoons/60ml olive oil
+ salt and pepper

Let's dive right into one of my favorite veggie starters, inspired by a recipe by Yotam Ottolenghi. You'll notice here that we're adding some cheese to it for taste—is that okay? Yes! Adding some protein or fat to our veggie starter is absolutely fine and does not reduce the power of the fiber in our veggies.

How to make it:

● Preheat the oven to 425°F. Place the chopped **cauliflower** and leaves in a roasting pan, toss them with 2 tablespoons of the **olive oil**, and season with **salt** and **pepper**. Pop the roasting pan in the oven and roast the cauliflower for 25 minutes, tossing halfway through.

● Meanwhile, make a dressing. In a small bowl, mix together the remaining 2 tablespoons of olive oil along with the **Dijon mustard** and **apple cider vinegar**. Season with salt and pepper.

● When the cauliflower is fork-tender, remove it from the oven and scatter the **Cheddar** and chopped **parsley** all over the top. Drizzle with the dressing and serve.

TIP: Toasted hazelnuts make a nice addition here, and you can team this with some grilled chicken for a lovely main meal.

Makes: 1 portion / Prep time: 10 min / Total cook time: 25 min
GLUTEN-FREE, VEGETARIAN

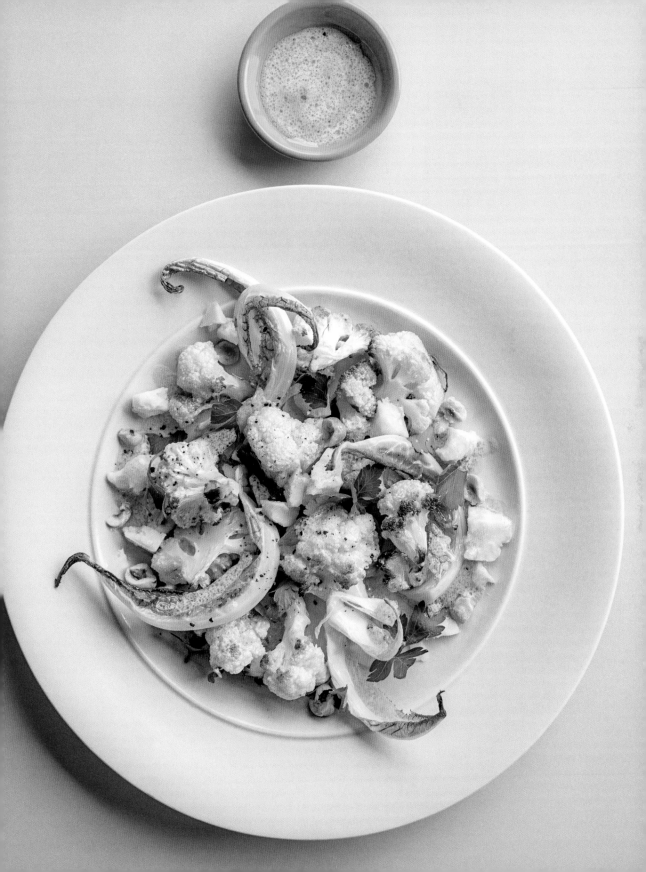

My cousin's MISO SPINACH

What you need:

2 teaspoons tahini

1 teaspoon white or brown miso

1 teaspoon soy sauce (or tamari, if you're gluten-free)

juice of ½ lemon

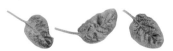

a large handful (about 2½ ounces/75g) of spinach

+ salt and pepper

My cousin Arthur's fresh spinach with miso dressing makes miso, I mean *me so*, excited that he has allowed me to share the recipe with you. The miso dressing boasts a tangy flavor, while still allowing the cool spinach to be the star of the show. This is the veggie starter of our dreams. And one of my absolute favorites in this book. Warning: very addictive.

How to make it:

● In a bowl, mix the **tahini, miso, soy sauce (or tamari),** and **lemon juice** together with 2 teaspoons of **water** until smooth and creamy.

● Tip the **spinach** into a serving bowl and pour the dressing over the top. Toss the leaves in the dressing and season them with **salt** and **pepper**. Enjoy your new favorite veggie starter!

Makes: 1 portion / Prep time: 5 min
GLUTEN-FREE **(if using tamari),** VEGAN

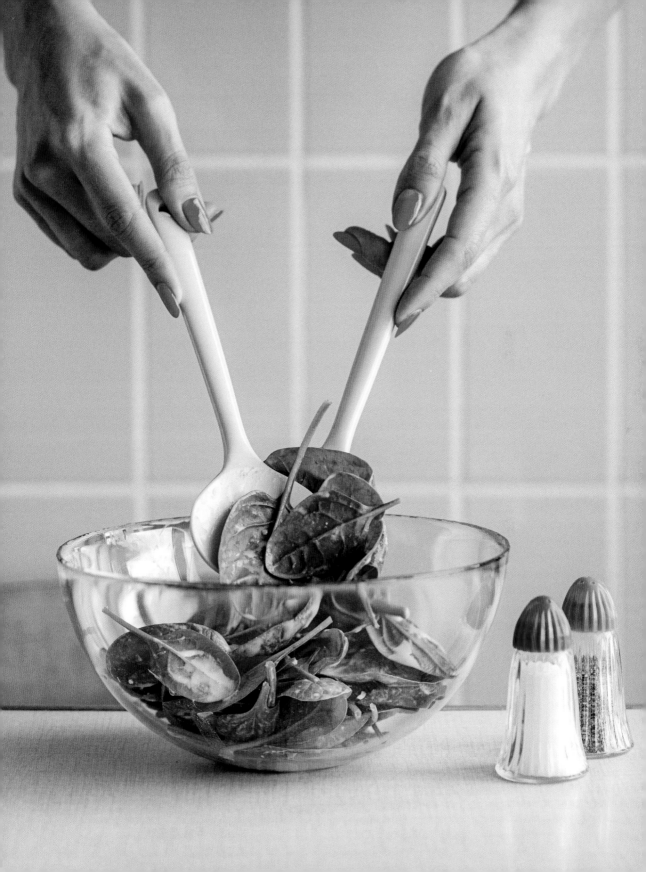

PEANUT BROCCOLI

What you need:

1 teaspoon soy sauce
(or tamari, if you're
gluten-free)

1 teaspoon sriracha

1 teaspoon unsweetened
peanut butter (make
sure the ingredients
are 100% peanuts)

1 teaspoon warm water

6–7 stalks of longstem
broccoli, tough ends
trimmed

chopped nuts of your choice
(optional)

Broccoli is a top contender in the world of veggie starters because of its very high fiber content. With its peanut butter dressing (yes, for real!), this recipe will surprise your taste buds and delight your glucose.

How to make it:

● In a small bowl, whisk together the **soy sauce (or tamari)**, **sriracha**, **peanut butter**, and **warm water** with a fork. It may look broken at first, but keep whisking and it will become smooth.

● Meanwhile, bring a small saucepan of water to a boil on high heat. Add the **broccoli** and blanch it for 2 minutes, to soften it briefly. Drain the broccoli and transfer it to a serving plate.

● Drizzle the dressing all over the broccoli and serve. Sprinkle with some chopped nuts for texture, if you have them on hand.

Makes: 1 portion / Prep time: 3 min / Total cook time: 3 min
GLUTEN-FREE (if using tamari), VEGAN

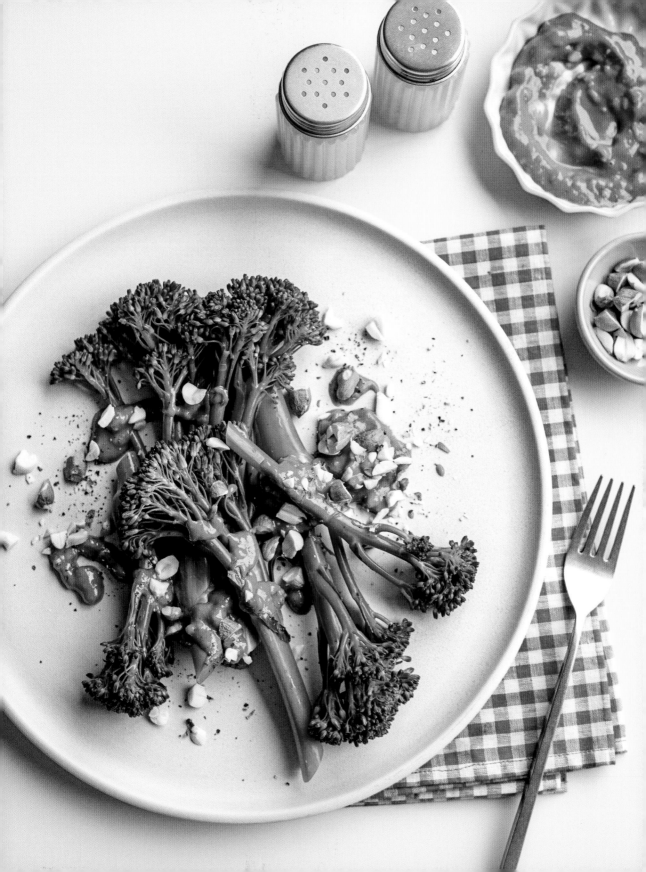

Beautiful batch of
ROASTED VEGGIES

What you need:

1 small eggplant, cut into ¾-inch/2cm chunks

1 red bell pepper, seeded and cut into ¾-inch/2cm chunks

1 small red onion, peeled and roughly sliced

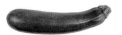

1 small zucchini, sliced into ¾-inch/2cm rounds

1 tablespoon basil pesto

a small handful of nuts, such as walnuts

+ 2 tablespoons olive oil
+ salt and pepper

One top community tip to make veggie starters easier is to cook them in batches in advance. So here is a simple recipe that provides four portions for you to keep in the fridge and whip out before meals. Easy!

How to make it:

● Preheat the oven to 425°F and line a large roasting pan with parchment paper.

● Spread **all the prepared veggies** in the pan. Drizzle with the **olive oil** and toss the vegetables to coat. Season with **salt** and **pepper**.

● Roast the vegetables in the oven for 20–25 minutes, tossing halfway through cooking, until nicely charred.

● Place a few heaping spoonfuls of the veggies into a serving bowl and add the **basil pesto**. Stir to coat, then top the veggies with the **nuts**.

● Save the leftover vegetables for the next few days. They will keep for 3–4 days stored in an airtight container in the fridge.

Makes: 4 portions / Prep time: 8 min / Total cook time: 25 min
GLUTEN-FREE, VEGETARIAN

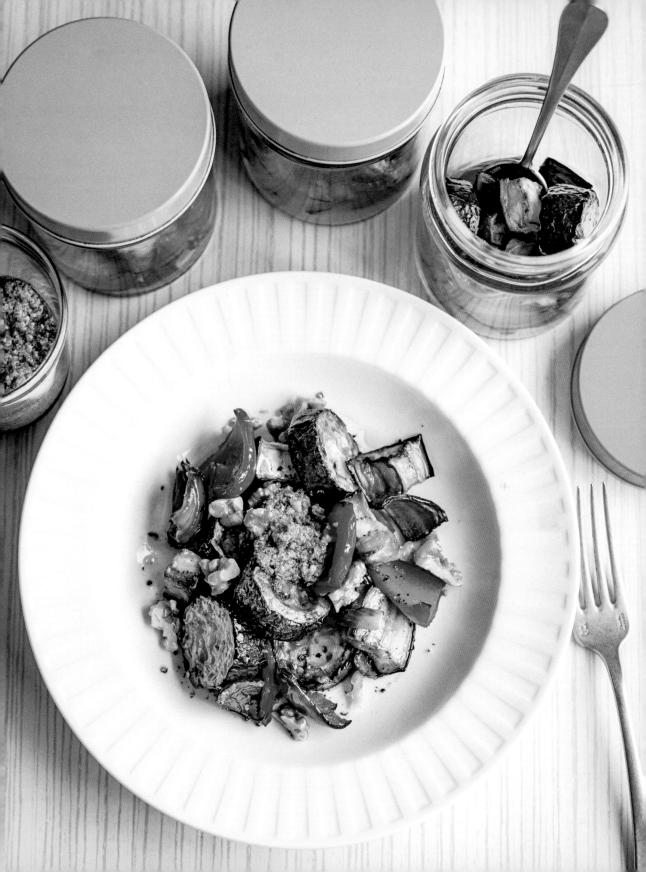

The GUMBALL MACHINE

COUNTS AS YOUR VINEGAR HACK FOR THE DAY AS WELL

What you need:

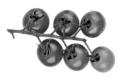

7 cherry tomatoes, halved

7 mini balls of mozzarella (bocconcini)

½ avocado, pitted and cut into chunks or balled

1 tablespoon balsamic vinegar

+ 1 tablespoon olive oil
+ salt and pepper

This is one of the very first veggie starters I ever put together and has remained a firm favorite. Extra points for how pretty and exciting to eat it is.

How to make it:

● Arrange the halved **tomatoes**, **mozzarella** balls, and chunks or balls of **avocado** in a bowl and drizzle the **balsamic vinegar** and **olive oil** all over. Season well with **salt** and **pepper**, and serve.

Makes: 1 portion / Prep time: 5 min
GLUTEN-FREE, VEGETARIAN

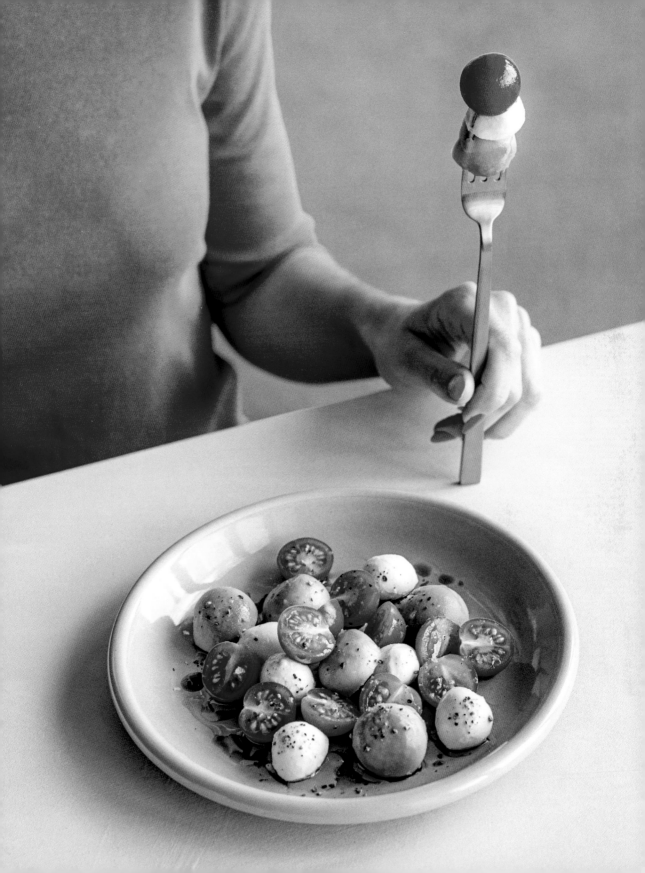

CHIMICHURRI CAULIFLOWER

What you need:

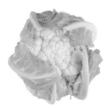

½ **small cauliflower, cut into florets (use the leaves, too)**

a small handful of flat-leaf parsley

a small handful of cilantro

1 teaspoon dried oregano

1 teaspoon sweet paprika (or any you have on hand)

juice of ½ lemon

+ **2 tablespoons olive oil**
+ **salt and pepper**

Here is cauliflower again, a wonderful fibrous vehicle for some delicious chimichurri sauce—and you'll have sauce left over for your other days. Picture the protective mesh from this veggie starting to reduce your glucose spike, and marvel at how you feel.

How to make it:

● Preheat the oven to 400°F and line a roasting pan with parchment paper. Lay the **cauliflower** florets and leaves in the roasting pan, then roast the cauliflower in the oven for 20–25 minutes, until tender.

● Meanwhile, make a chimichurri dressing. Place the **parsley, cilantro, oregano, paprika, lemon juice**, and **olive oil** in a mini food processor and blitz the mixture until smooth. (Alternatively, finely chop the fresh herbs and then stir them into the dried orgeano, paprika, lemon juice, and olive oil.) Season the dressing well with **salt** and **pepper**.

● When the cauliflower is ready, transfer it to a serving dish and drizzle with half of the chimichurri dressing, then serve.

● Transfer the remaining chimichurri dressing to a small airtight jar. It will keep in the fridge for up to 5 days and is delicious drizzled over any roast veg.

Makes: 1 portion / Prep time: 8 min / Total cook time: 25 min
GLUTEN-FREE, VEGAN

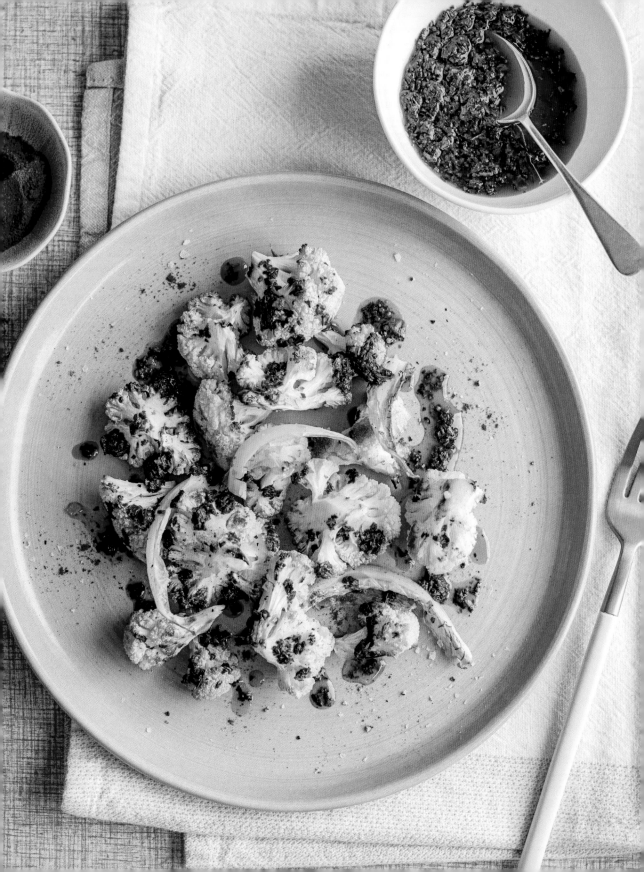

BITTER LEAF SALAD *with* YOGURT DRESSING

What you need:

1 tablespoon full-fat Greek yogurt

juice of ½ lemon

2 tablespoons finely grated Parmesan

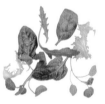

2 handfuls of mixed lettuce leaves

a small handful of blanched hazelnuts (optional)

+ 1 tablespoon olive oil
+ salt and pepper

"Sure, I'm a little bitter, but at least I'm well-dressed" would likely be the tagline in this salad's online dating profile. Swipe right! Take a chance and go on a date with this veggie starter. I'm sure you'll get along beautifully.

How to make it:

● In a bowl, mix the **yogurt**, **lemon juice**, **Parmesan**, and **olive oil** together to make a dressing and season it with **salt** and **pepper**.

● Tip the **lettuce leaves** into a serving bowl and drizzle with the dressing. Toss the leaves until they are thoroughly coated, then sprinkle with the hazelnuts, if using, and serve.

Makes: 1 portion / Prep time: 8 min
GLUTEN-FREE, VEGETARIAN

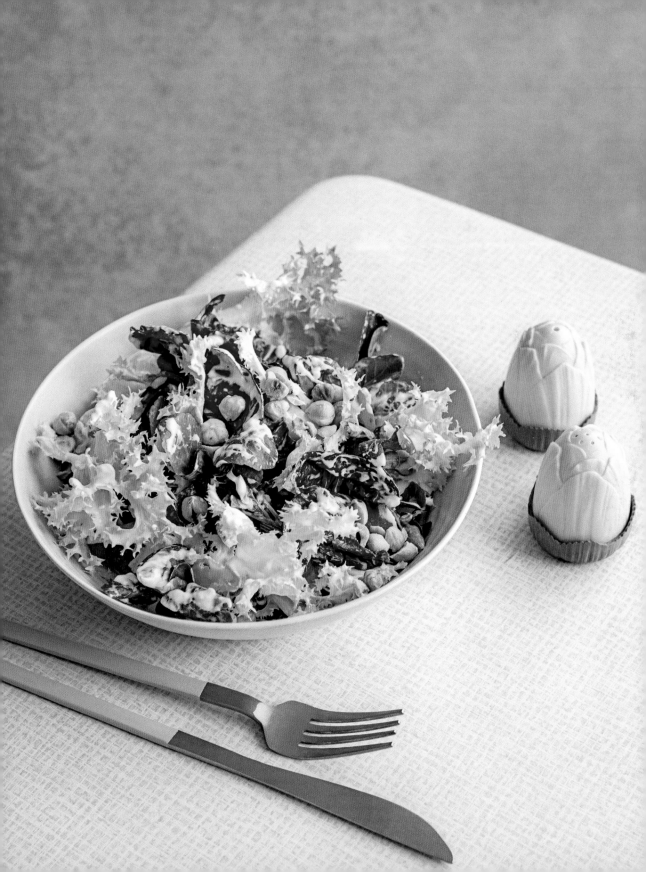

CHARRED BRUSSELS SPROUTS *with* BACON *and* TOASTED HAZELNUTS

What you need:

2 slices of bacon, cut into small pieces

12 Brussels sprouts, halved

3 tablespoons roughly chopped hazelnuts, blanched if you prefer

a squeeze of lemon juice

+ 1½ tablespoons olive oil
+ salt and pepper

You had me at bacon.

How to make it:

● Drizzle ½ tablespoon of the **olive oil** into a medium frying pan and place the pan on medium heat. Add the chopped **bacon** and fry for 3 minutes, until the pieces are browned and crispy. Remove the bacon from the pan, leaving behind the rendered fat, and set the bacon aside.

● Add the **Brussels sprouts** to the pan and turn up the heat. Fry the sprouts for about 10 minutes, tossing them regularly, until they are nicely charred. Return the bacon to the pan and heat everything through. Then tip everything into a serving bowl or onto a plate.

● Top the sprout and bacon mixture with the **hazelnuts**, drizzle with a squeeze of **lemon juice**, and finish with the remaining olive oil. Season with **salt** and **pepper**, and serve.

Makes: 1 portion / Prep time: 8 min / Total cook time: 15 min
GLUTEN-FREE

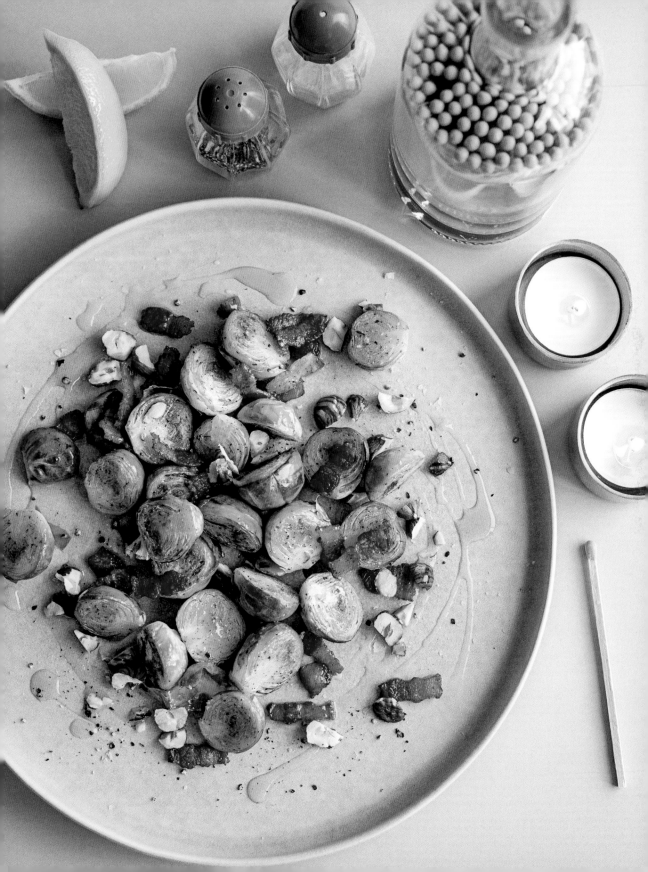

FRENCHIE ASPARAGUS

COUNTS AS YOUR VINEGAR HACK FOR THE DAY AS WELL

What you need:

2 teaspoons Dijon mustard

1 tablespoon vinegar (any kind)

1 jar of white asparagus, drained (about 7 ounces/ 200g, drained weight)

+ 2 teaspoons olive oil
+ salt and pepper

Bonjour! So many cousins, so little space to share all their recipes. This is another family favorite passed on to me by a relative. The Frenchie Asparagus's simple prep and surprising burst of flavor make it a go-to veggie starter. No cooking involved, *and* it counts as your vinegar for the day. *Oui, oui. Merci beaucoup!*

How to make it:

● In a small bowl, whisk together the **mustard**, **vinegar**, and **olive oil** with a fork until they have emulsified to make a dressing. Season with **salt** and **pepper**.

● Arrange the **white asparagus** on a plate, drizzle the dressing all over the top, and season to taste with salt and pepper. Serve and enjoy!

Makes: 1 portion / Prep time: 5 min
GLUTEN-FREE, VEGAN

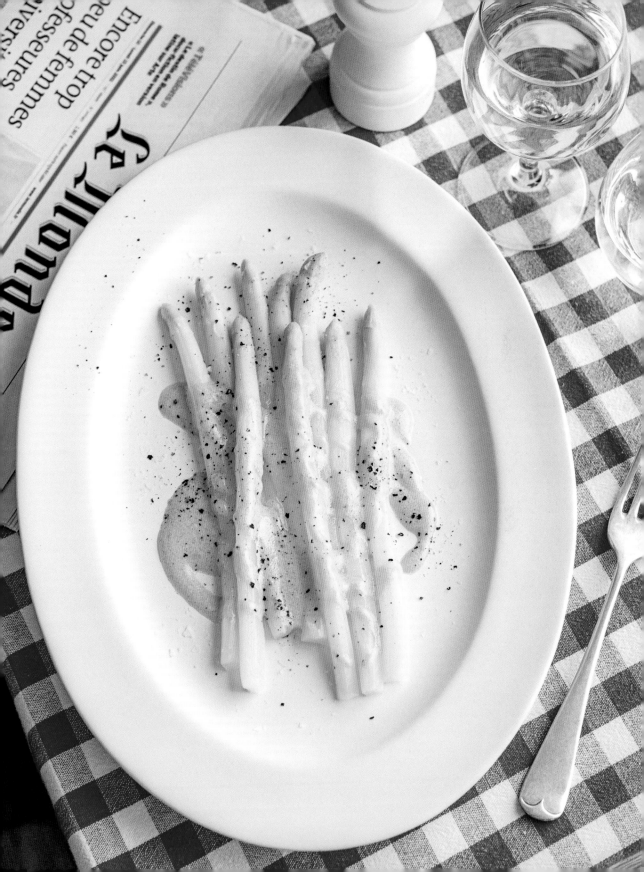

BACKWARD BROCCOLI

What you need:

¼ head of broccoli, finely
   chopped
boiling water

3 tablespoons full-fat Greek
yogurt

1½ teaspoons harissa paste

+ salt and pepper

We have all thrown raw veggies into boiling water, but have you ever poured boiling water into a bowl of raw broccoli? Didn't think so. This might be one of those things you have to see to believe, so get out the kettle and get boiling.

How to make it:

● Place the **broccoli** in a heatproof bowl and cover it with **boiling water**. Set the bowl aside for 2 minutes to soften the veg.

● Meanwhile, spread the **yogurt** on a serving plate and mix in the **harissa**.

● Drain the broccoli, then scatter it all over the harissa yogurt. Season generously with **salt** and **pepper**, and serve.

Makes: 1 portion / Prep time: 5 min / Total cook time: 2 min
GLUTEN-FREE, VEGETARIAN

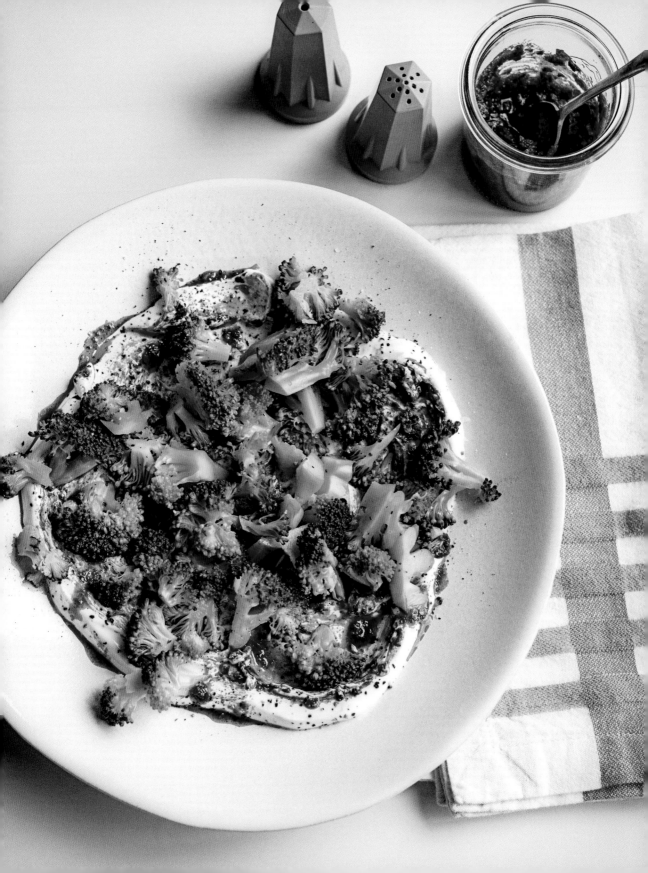

TAHINI GREENS

What you need:

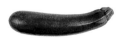

½ **zucchini, halved lengthwise and thinly sliced into half moons**

a small handful of sugar snap peas, roughly chopped

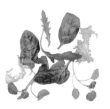

a handful of mixed lettuce leaves

1 tablespoon tahini

juice of ½ lemon

1 tablespoon ice-cold water

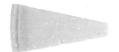

2 tablespoons coarsely grated Parmesan

+ salt and pepper

A little tahini, a bowl full of greeny, keeps me from feeling like a total meanie. Don't take that rhyme as a hint that my next book will feature poetry. It won't. But one thing I will be doing is whipping up this bowl of goodness as my next veggie starter. Throw whatever greens you have on hand into a big bowl, from Brussels sprouts to lettuce, or green beans or even peas. Top them with this tasty tahini dressing and some grated Parmesan. Yum!

How to make it:

● In a serving bowl, toss the sliced **zucchini**, chopped **sugar snap peas,** and the **lettuce** together.

● In a separate, small bowl, mix the **tahini** and **lemon juice** together with the **ice-cold water** to make a dressing. Season with **salt** and **pepper** and drizzle the dressing all over the greens.

● Sprinkle the **Parmesan** over the top, season the salad with salt and pepper, and serve.

Makes: 1 portion / Prep time: 10 min
GLUTEN-FREE, VEGETARIAN

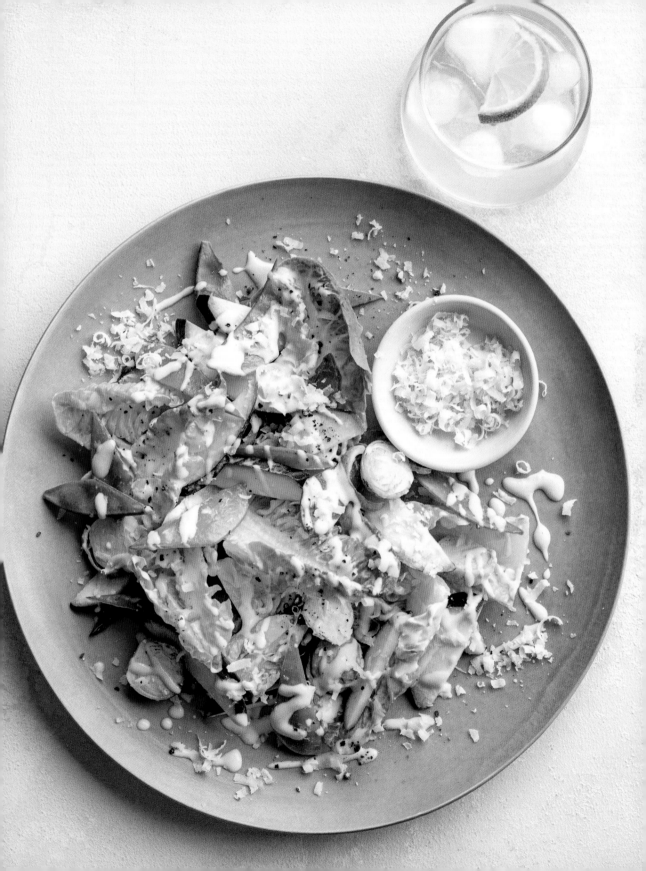

Fridge RATATOUILLE

What you need:

1 red onion,
roughly chopped

1 eggplant, cut into
¾-inch/2cm chunks

3 garlic cloves,
roughly
chopped

3 bell peppers (use a mixture
of colors), seeded
and roughly chopped

1 x 14-ounce/400g can of
chopped tomatoes

2 tablespoons
balsamic
vinegar

+ 2 tablespoons olive oil
+ salt and pepper

Top tip from the wonderful people who completed the Glucose Goddess Method before you: cook batches of veggie starters in advance and keep them in the fridge until you're ready to eat. Well, here's another recipe perfectly suited to that plan. This recipe makes four portions, *and* it's a great "take to work" veggie starter. Just a note: while you see balsamic vinegar used here, there isn't enough vinegar in total in the recipe to count as your vinegar hack for the day.

How to make it:

• Heat the **olive oil** in a medium saucepan on medium heat. Add the chopped **red onion** and **eggplant** chunks and fry them for 2 minutes. Add the chopped **garlic** and fry for 30 seconds more, to soften.

• Add the chunks of **bell pepper**, the chopped **tomatoes**, and **balsamic vinegar**. Stir everything together, then bring the liquid to a simmer. Cover and cook the ratatouille on high heat for 15 minutes, stirring from time to time, until the vegetables are soft.

• Season the ratatouille with **salt** and **pepper**, then let it cool and transfer it to an airtight container. It will keep for up to 5 days in the fridge.

Makes: 4 portions / Prep time: 10 min / Total cook time: 20 min
GLUTEN-FREE, VEGAN

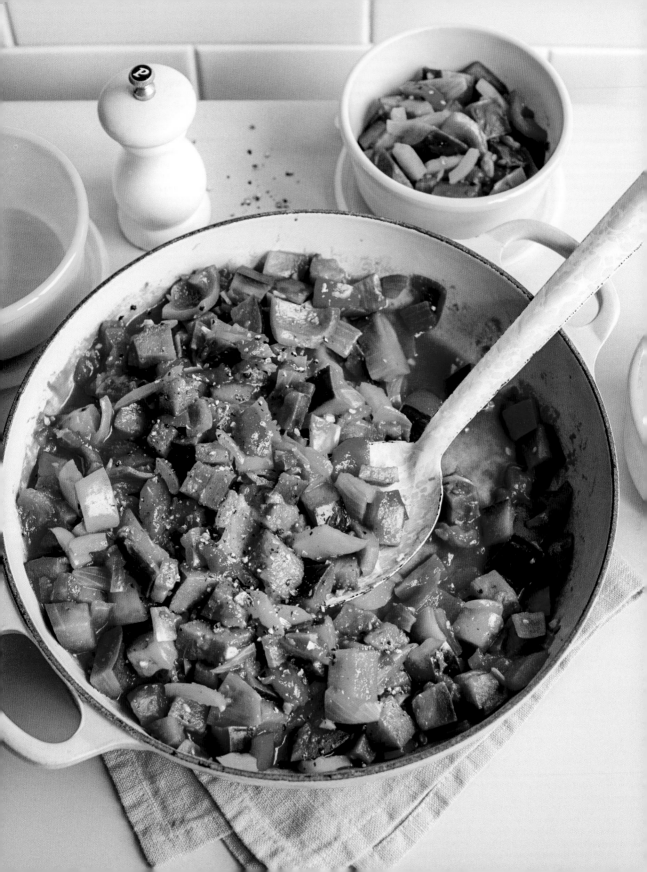

No-teeth BEAN PUREE

What you need:

¾ cup/100g frozen fava beans

1 garlic clove

zest and juice of ½ large unwaxed lemon

+ 2 tablespoons olive oil
+ salt and pepper

No teeth, no problem. While it is best to consume our veggies whole (blending reduces the power of the fiber they contain), there are some occasions when something sippable is just what we need. This puree also makes a great dip, served with radishes or mixed veg crudités.

How to make it:

● Bring a small saucepan of water to a boil on high heat, then lower the heat and let the water calm to a simmer. Add the **frozen fava beans** and **garlic clove** to the pan and simmer for 1 minute, until the fava beans have softened.

● Drain the beans and garlic and transfer them to a deep bowl. Add the **olive oil** and **lemon zest** and **juice**. Using an immersion blender, blitz the mixture until it's smooth. Season with **salt** and **pepper**.

Makes: 1 portion / Prep time: 5 min / Total cook time: 1 min
GLUTEN-FREE, VEGAN

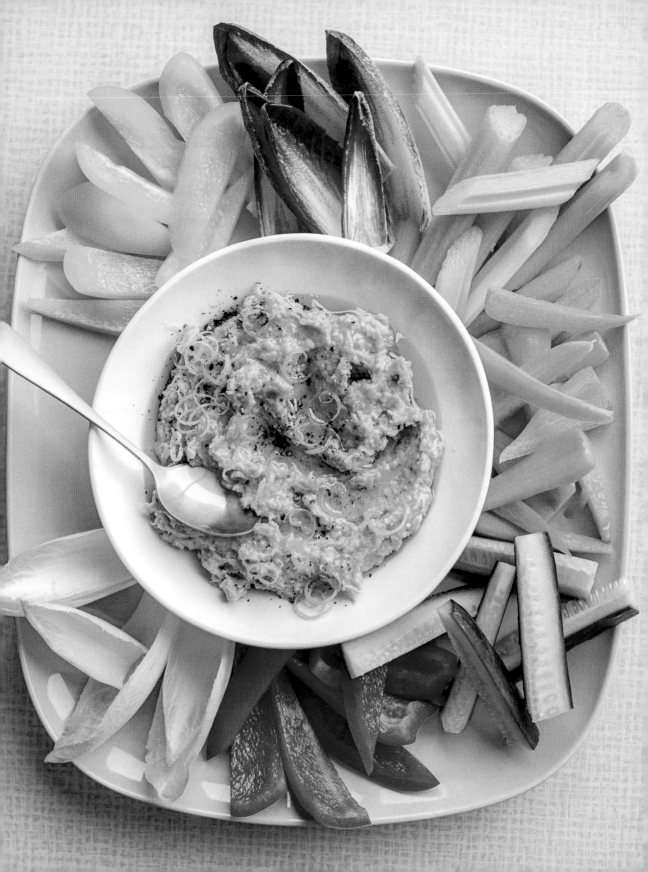

Fancy ZUCCHINI ROLLS
to share

What you need:

¼ cup/60g ricotta

2 tablespoons finely grated Parmesan

1¾ ounces/50g frozen spinach, defrosted and excess water squeezed out

1 teaspoon ground nutmeg

1 tablespoon pine nuts, toasted

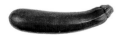

1 small zucchini, sliced lengthwise into ribbons with a mandoline or peeler

+ salt and pepper

Top tip when making this recipe: make sure to get all that excess liquid out of the spinach. Squeeze it between your hands—you will be amazed at how much comes out. What's left is all the fiber! Which is what we're after. The ricotta filling for these rolls also doubles as a delicious pasta sauce, finished with a squeeze of lemon. Scale the recipe up if you're feeding a crowd.

How to make it:

• Make the filling. In a bowl, mix together the **ricotta**, **Parmesan**, squeezed **spinach**, **nutmeg**, and toasted **pine nuts** and season generously with **salt** and **pepper**.

• Lay out the ribbons of **zucchini** and spread equal amounts of the filling mixture along the length of each. Roll up each filled ribbon into a spiral. Arrange the spirals on a serving plate, and serve.

Makes: 2 portions / Prep time: 15 min
GLUTEN-FREE, VEGETARIAN

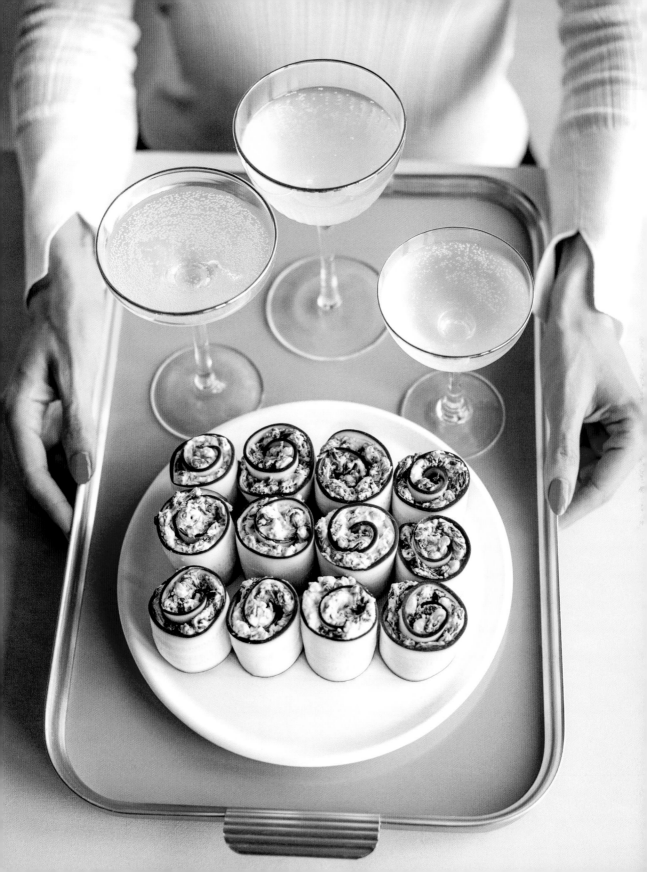

My aunt's
PURPLE RED CABBAGE SALAD

What you need:

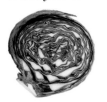

¼ **small red cabbage,
finely sliced**

juice of ½ lemon

**a small handful of
pomegranate seeds
(about 2 tablespoons)**

**5–6 cilantro sprigs, stems
trimmed, leaves roughly
chopped**

**+ 1 tablespoon olive oil
+ salt and pepper**

If I keep stealing recipes from my relatives, this book is going to start reading more like a family tree than a cookbook. Maybe that's okay. Anyway, this cabbage salad is not only pleasing on the palate, it's total eye candy, too. The bright purples and deep reds from the cabbage and pomegranate seeds make it look like a work of art! A great veggie starter choice when hosting or cooking for others, especially since it's so easy to scale up.

How to make it:

● In a bowl, toss the sliced **cabbage** with the **lemon juice** and **olive oil**, then add the **pomegranate seeds** and chopped **cilantro** and stir to combine. Season with **salt** and **pepper**, and serve.

Makes: 1 portion / Prep time: 10 min
GLUTEN-FREE, VEGAN

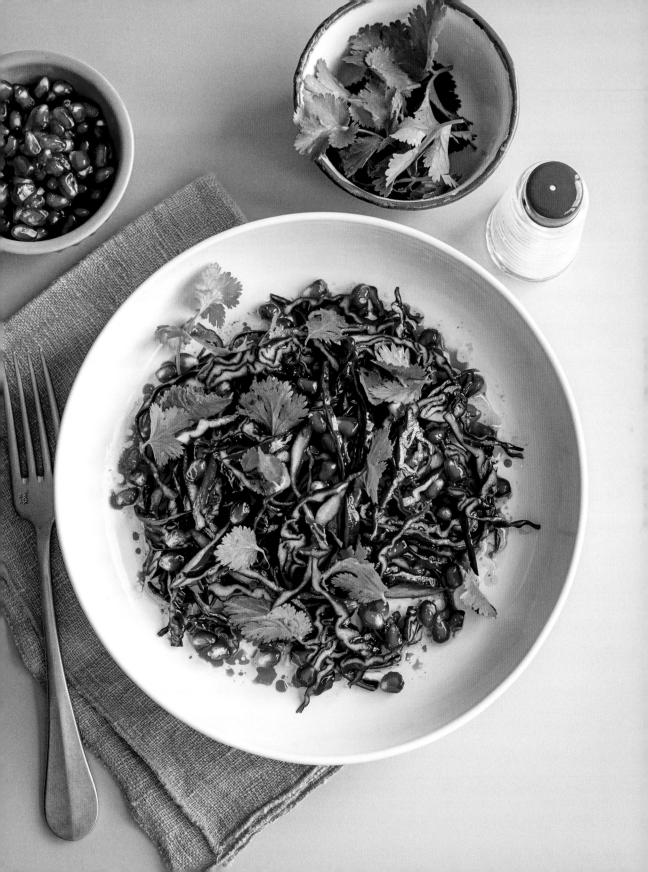

HOT ROMAINE

What you need:

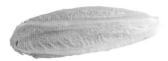

1 head of romaine lettuce, halved lengthwise

+ 1 tablespoon olive oil

+ salt and pepper

I thought my love of cool, crunchy lettuce leaves ran deep . . . and then I tried grilling them. Absolute veggie starter game changer. This recipe requires only one main ingredient, the romaine itself, and a few other items you're sure to have on hand. An excellent option when you're short on groceries, time, or both!

How to make it:

● Heat the **olive oil** in a griddle pan or large frying pan on high heat.

● Once the oil is hot, add the **romaine lettuce** halves to the pan, cut sides down, and grill them for 2 minutes, until the undersides are starting to brown. Carefully turn over the lettuce halves and grill the other sides for another 2 minutes.

● Season generously with **salt** and **pepper** and transfer to a plate to serve.

Makes: 1 portion / Prep time: 2 min / Total cook time: 4 min
GLUTEN-FREE, VEGAN

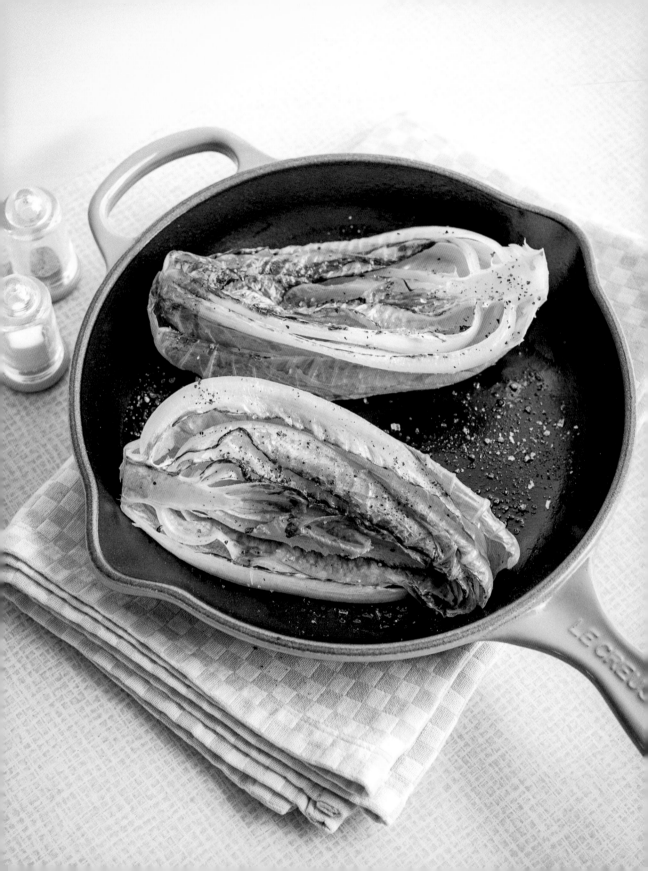

BABY RADISHES *with* DILL *and* YOGURT

What you need:

12 radishes, halved

1 tablespoon full-fat Greek yogurt

5–6 dill sprigs, stems trimmed, leaves finely chopped

+ 1 tablespoon olive oil
+ salt and pepper

A community favorite, this veggie starter is as easy to assemble as it is amazing for your taste buds. A great one, too, if you have little ones at home who want to jump on the veggie starter train.

How to make it:

● In a serving bowl, place the halved **radishes**, **Greek yogurt**, chopped **dill**, and **olive oil** and toss them together to combine. Season the mixture generously with **salt** and **pepper**, then serve.

Makes: 2 portions / Prep time: 5 min
GLUTEN-FREE

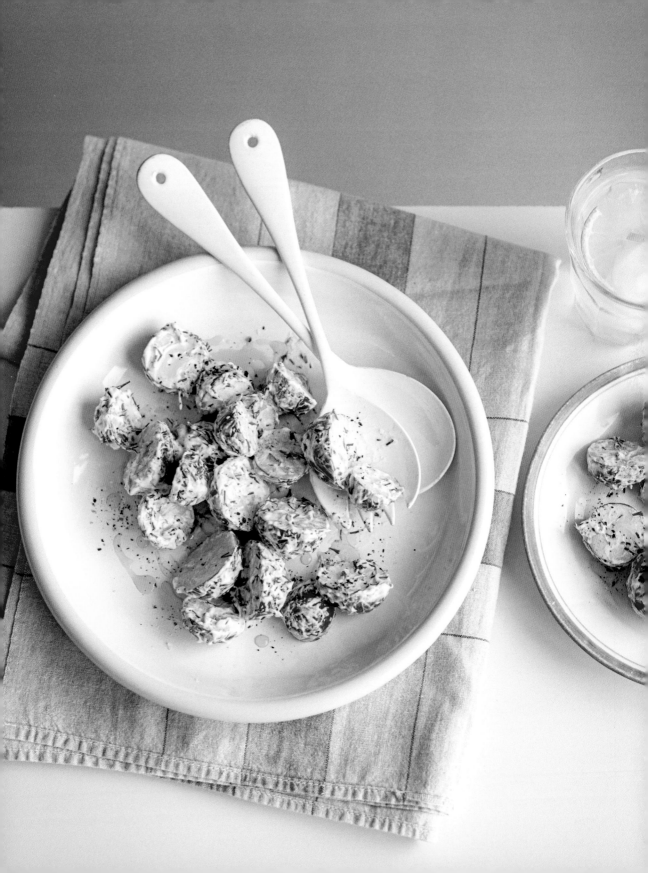

My mom's
SLOW-COOKED LEEKS

What you need:

a large knob of butter

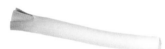

1 small leek, finely sliced

a small handful of flat-leaf parsley, stems trimmed, leaves roughly chopped

+ salt and pepper

Nothing says comfort quite like Mom's cooking. This one is for when you have lots of time to spare, because these leeks need a good 30 minutes to slowly caramelize in the pan. Worth the wait.

How to make it:

● Melt the **butter** in a medium frying pan on medium heat.

● Once melted, lower the heat to very low and add the sliced **leek**. Fry for 25–30 minutes, stirring from time to time, until soft and silky. Season the leek with **salt** and **pepper**, top with the chopped **parsley**, and serve.

Makes: 1 portion / Prep time: 5 min / Total cook time: 30 min
GLUTEN-FREE, VEGETARIAN

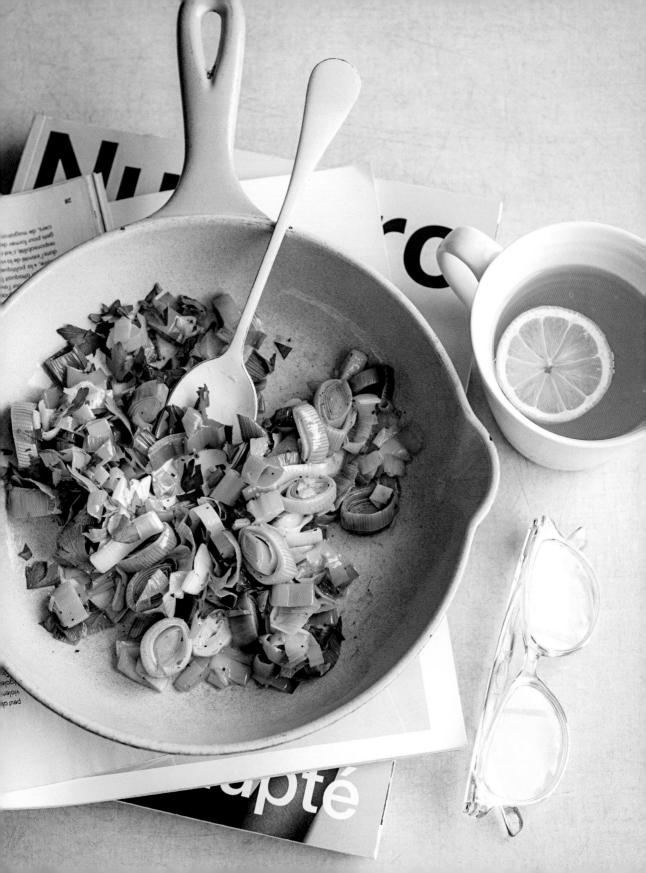

Sorry, more-Parmesan
GARLIC GREEN BEANS

What you need:

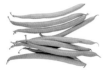

5¼ ounces/150g green beans, trimmed

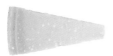

1 tablespoon softened butter

1 garlic clove, finely chopped or grated

2 tablespoons finely grated Parmesan

+ salt and pepper

Okay, I'm not *really* sorry. Of all the proteins and fats that we like adding to our veggie starters to make them tastier, Parmesan is unapologetically one of my favorites. A thing of beauty.

How to make it:

● Preheat the oven to 400°F and line a small roasting pan with parchment paper.

● In a bowl, toss the **green beans** with the softened **butter** and chopped or grated **garlic** until the beans are thoroughly coated.

● Tip out the beans in a single layer into the lined roasting pan and scatter the **Parmesan** all over.

● Season the beans with **salt** and **pepper** and roast them in the oven for 15 minutes, or until the cheese is golden and crispy. Serve.

Makes: 1 portion / Prep time: 5 min / Total cook time: 15 min
GLUTEN-FREE, VEGETARIAN

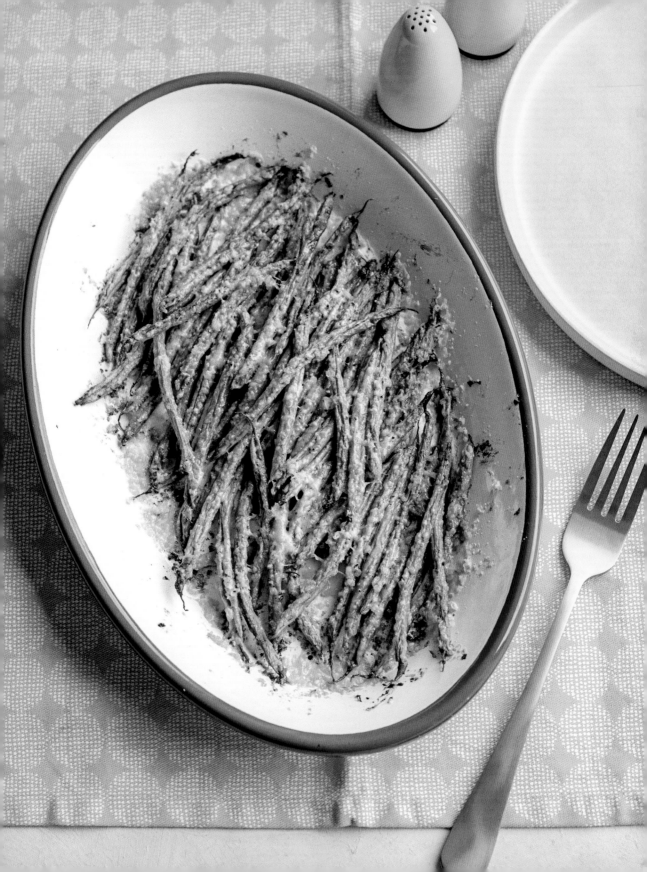

ZUCCHINI *with* ANCHOVIES

What you need:

a knob of butter

1 garlic clove, roughly chopped

1 zucchini, sliced into ½-inch/1cm rounds

2 anchovies, drained and roughly chopped

a small bunch of flat-leaf parsley, stems trimmed, leaves roughly chopped

lemon juice, to serve (optional)

+ salt and pepper

Another punchy way to add flavor to your veggie starter: anchovies! (Divisive, I know, but if you love them, this is for you.) They are fantastic for your health because of their high content of omega-3 fatty acids, which offers powerful benefits for your heart. Store a jar of anchovies in the fridge and use them in the same way on other greens, such as chopped broccoli, sliced cabbage, or Brussels sprouts.

How to make it:

• Melt the **butter** in a frying pan on medium heat. Once melted, add the chopped **garlic** and sliced **zucchini** and fry them for 5–7 minutes, until softened and slightly browned.

• Stir in the chopped **anchovies** and cook for 1 minute more.

• Remove the pan from the heat. Add the chopped **parsley**, and season with **salt** and **pepper**. Serve with a squeeze of lemon juice, if you have any fresh lemons on hand.

Makes: 1 portion / Prep time: 8 min / Total cook time: 8 min
GLUTEN-FREE

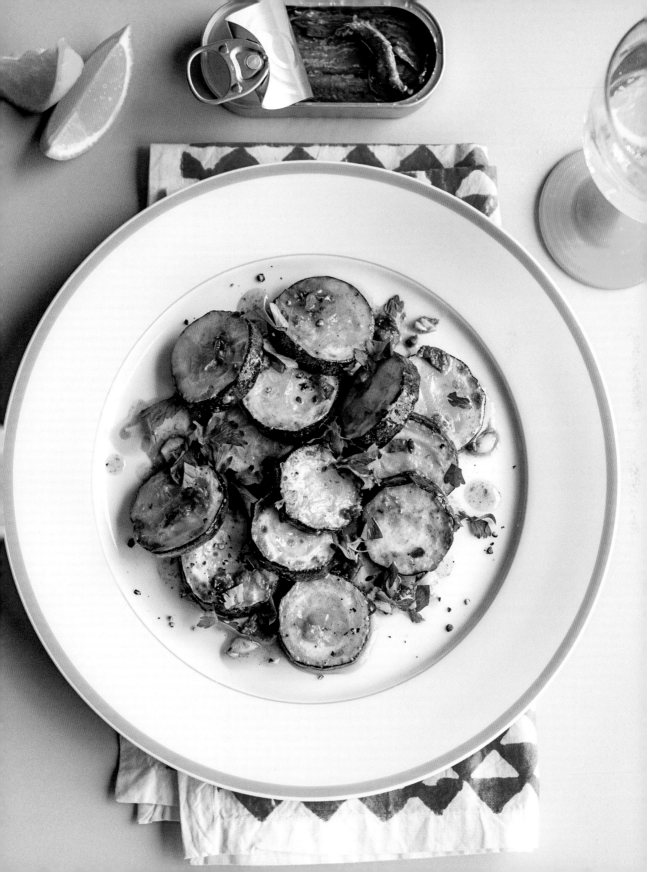

BAKED FENNEL

What you need:

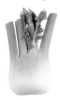

1 fennel bulb, trimmed and cut into wedges

½ lemon, cut into wedges

about 10 pitted green olives, halved

+ 1 tablespoon olive oil
+ salt and pepper

If you've never baked fennel, this is your sign to try it out. A top-tier veggie starter.

How to make it:

● Preheat the oven to 400°F. Place the **fennel** wedges, **lemon** wedges, and **olive** halves in a roasting dish, drizzle them with the **olive oil**, and season them with **salt** and **pepper**.

● Bake for 20 minutes, until the fennel is softened and beginning to char, then remove the dish from the oven and allow everything to cool slightly. Squeeze out some of the juice from the roasted lemon wedges onto the roasted fennel, and serve.

Makes: 1 portion / Prep time: 5 min / Total cook time: 20 min
GLUTEN-FREE, VEGAN

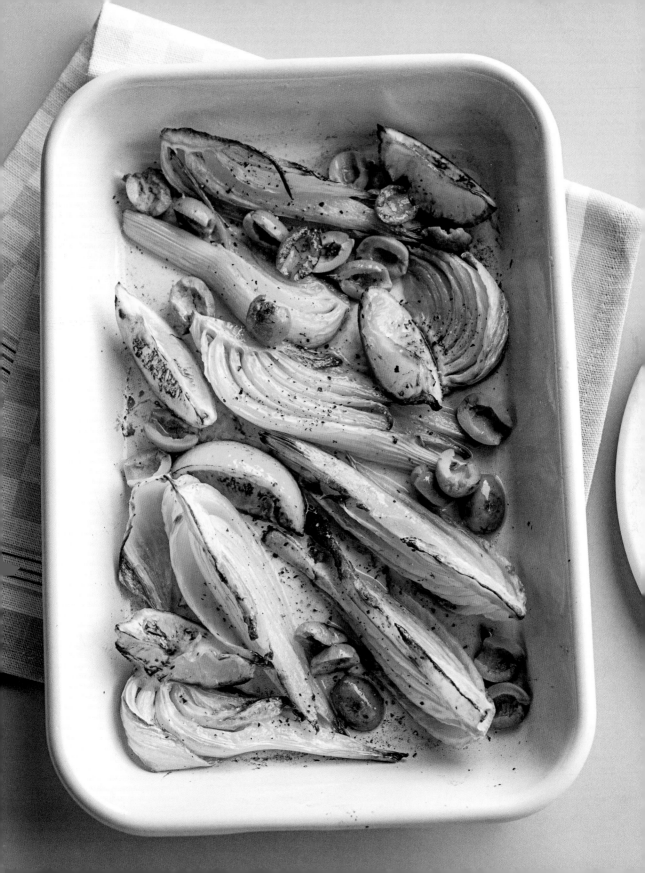

5-MIN SOUP

What you need:

1¾ ounces/50g frozen spinach

¼ small broccoli head (about 3½ ounces/100g), finely chopped

1¼ cups/300ml boiling water

1 tablespoon white or brown miso

1 tablespoon soy sauce (or tamari, if you're gluten-free)

juice of ½ lime

I haven't checked the *Guinness Book of World Records* yet, so I can't be completely sure, but this has to be one of the fastest soups to prepare of all-time. And also one of the best soups for our veggie starter mission because the veggies in it are still whole (not blended)—so the fiber is intact. Ready, steady, go!

How to make it:

● Place the **frozen spinach** and the chopped **broccoli** in a medium saucepan with the **boiling water**. Place the pan on high heat with the lid on and bring the water back to a boil for about 45 seconds, until the vegetables are cooked. Remove the pan from the heat.

● Stir in the **miso**, **soy sauce or tamari**, and **lime juice**, and serve.

Makes: 1 portion / Prep time: 5 min / Total cook time: 5 min
GLUTEN-FREE (if using tamari), VEGAN

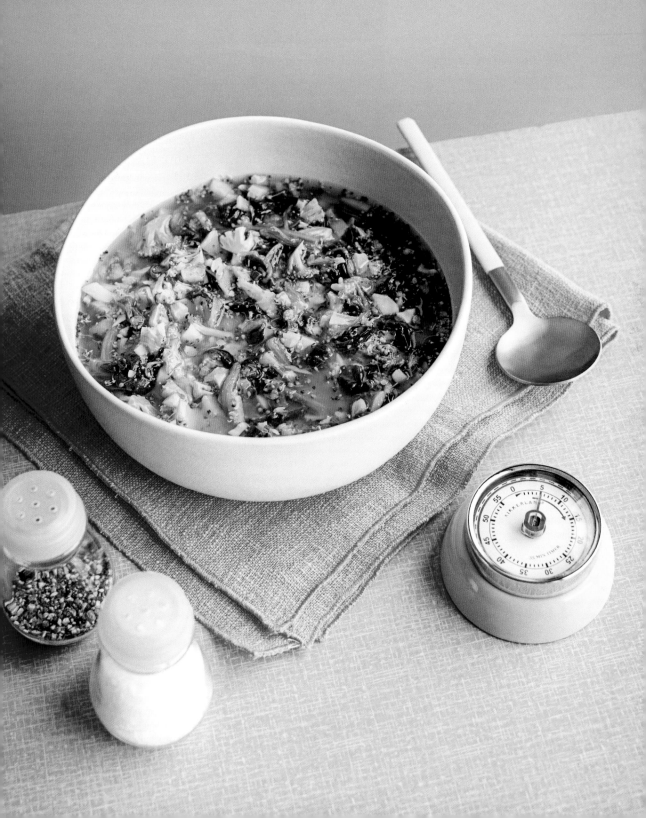

CRISPY KALE

What you need:

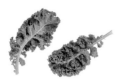

1 bunch kale, stems removed and sliced (or use precut)

½–1 teaspoon chile flakes (depending on how spicy you like your food!)

+ 1 tablespoon olive oil
+ salt and pepper

If you've turned up your nose at kale before, take another chance on it using this recipe. The chile flakes add a pop of heat, while oven-baking the kale reduces some of the bite in it that can sometimes be off-putting. A dreamy veggie starter that is also excellent made in advance and enjoyed cold.

How to make it:

● Preheat the oven to 400°F. Place the **kale** slices in a roasting dish, drizzle them with the **olive oil**, then sprinkle with the **chile flakes**. Season with **salt** and **pepper**.

● Use your hands to massage the oil into the kale so that it is thoroughly coated.

● Place the dish in the oven for 7 minutes, tossing the kale around a little halfway through cooking, until tender and slightly crisped at the edges. Serve then and there, or enjoy cold later on.

Makes: 1 portion / Prep time: 3 min / Total cook time: 7 min
GLUTEN-FREE, VEGAN

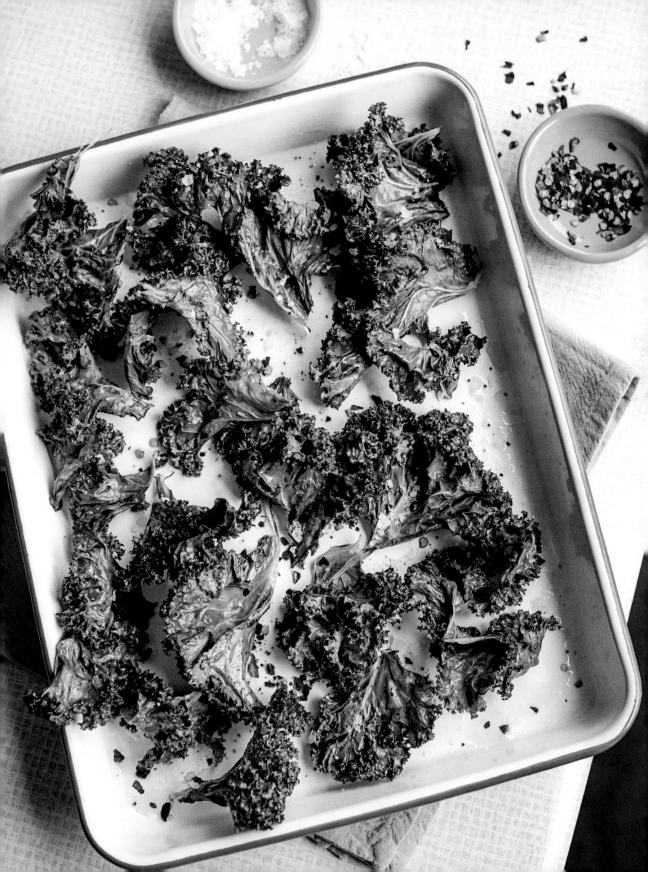

LAZY TZATZIKI

What you need:

½ **large cucumber, halved lengthwise, seeds scraped out, cut into chunks**

2 tablespoons full-fat Greek yogurt

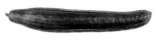

a large handful of mint, stemmed

+ **1 tablespoon olive oil**
+ **salt and pepper**

Working smart, not hard, is the name of the game in the Glucose Goddess Method. And this recipe is a great example: leave the mint leaves whole and keep the cucumber chunky.

How to make it:

● Place the **cucumber** chunks, **yogurt**, **mint** leaves, and **olive oil** in a bowl. Toss everything together to coat the cucumber. Season with **salt** and **pepper**, and serve.

Makes: 1 portion / Prep time: 5 min
GLUTEN-FREE, VEGETARIAN

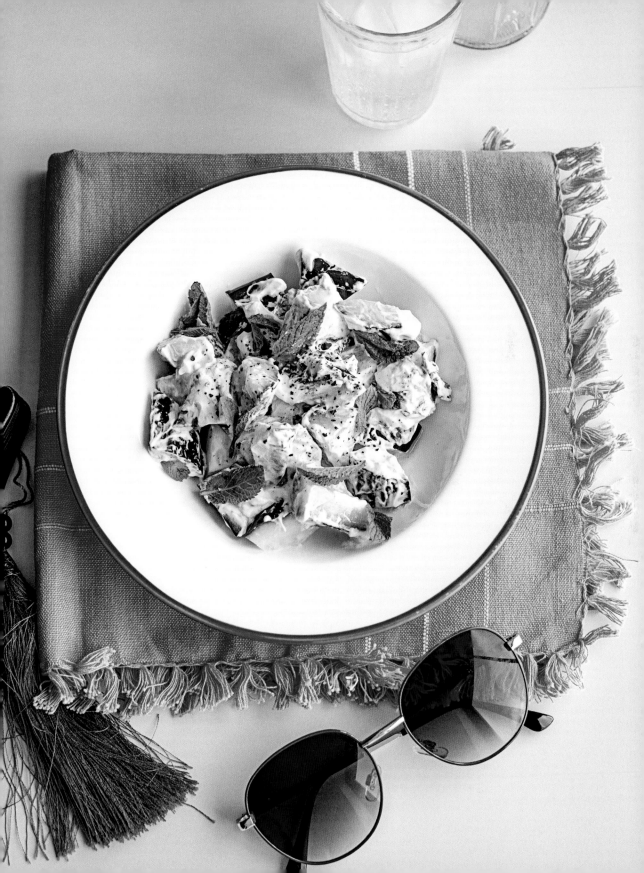

PARMESAN *and* BALSAMIC COUPLE

COUNTS AS YOUR VINEGAR HACK FOR THE DAY AS WELL

What you need:

a large handful of arugula

1 tablespoon balsamic vinegar

2 tablespoons finely grated or shaved Parmesan

+ 2 teaspoons olive oil
+ salt and pepper

There's a lot of debate in the food world about which pairing is the true dynamic duo. Peanut butter and jelly, grapes and cheese, and chocolate and more chocolate are some typical contenders, but if you ask me, Parmesan and balsamic are the greatest culinary couple there is.

How to make it:

● Toss the **arugula** in a bowl with the **balsamic vinegar** and **olive oil**. Season with **salt** and **pepper**, and sprinkle with the finely grated or shaved **Parmesan** to finish.

Makes: 1 portion / Prep time: 3 min
GLUTEN-FREE, VEGETARIAN

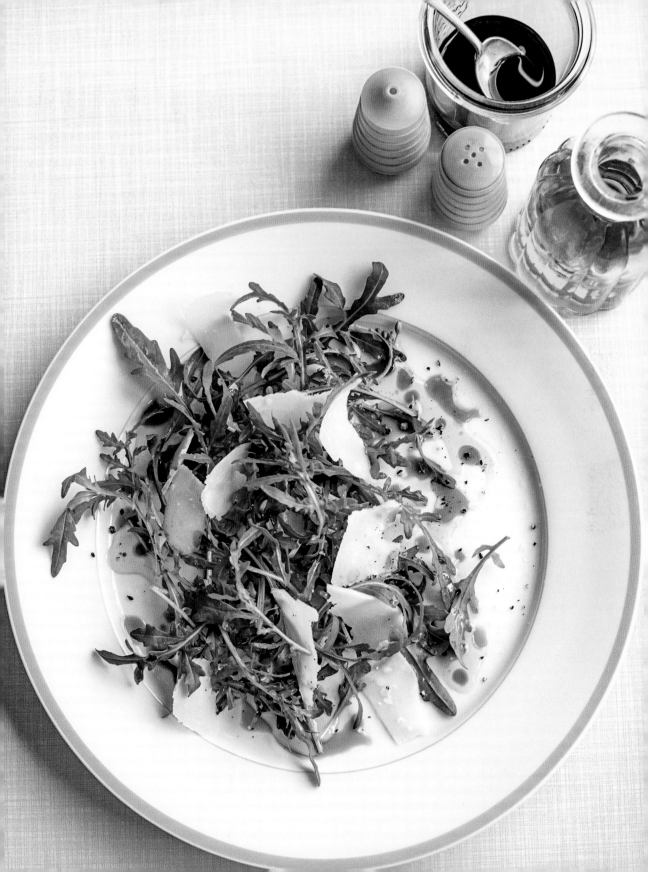

ARTICHOKE, PEA, LEMON, OLIVES

What you need:

half of 1 x 7-ounce/200g jar
of marinated artichokes in oil,
drained (about 3 ounces/80g
drained weight)

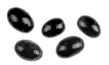

½ cup/80g frozen peas,
defrosted

8 pitted black olives, halved

zest and juice of ½ unwaxed
lemon

+ 1 tablespoon olive oil
+ salt and pepper

What did the lemon say to the artichokes and peas? I don't want olive you. Artichokes are an excellent choice of fibrous veggies, and here is an easy way to prepare them.

How to make it:

● In a bowl, arrange the **artichokes**, defrosted **peas**, and **olive** halves. Top with the **lemon zest** and **juice**, and drizzle with the **olive oil**. Season with **salt** and **pepper**, and serve.

Makes: 1 portion / Prep time: 8 min
GLUTEN-FREE, VEGAN

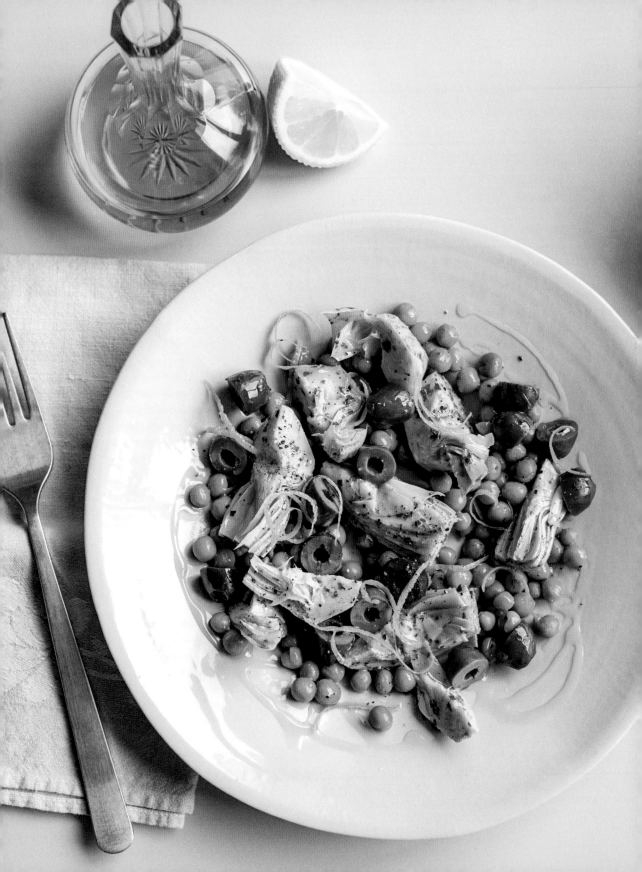

LOVER'S SALAD

What you need:

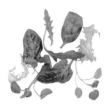

a handful of salad leaves
(of your choice)

6 cherry tomatoes, halved

6 cucumber slices

 5–6 dill or basil
sprigs, stemmed

 ½ ounce/
15g feta,
crumbled

1 teaspoon za'atar

juice of ½ lemon

+ 1 tablespoon olive oil
+ salt and pepper

I cannot confirm or deny whether this dish has single-handedly united a few couples. But if you've got your eye on someone special, maybe this is your prompt: double up this recipe and invite them over for dinner. Just saying.

How to make it:

● Arrange the **salad leaves**, halved **tomatoes**, slices of **cucumber**, **dill or basil** leaves, and crumbled **feta** on a plate.

● Sprinkle the **za'atar** all over, then add a generous squeeze of **lemon juice** and the **olive oil**. Season with **salt** and **pepper**, then stir everything together to combine and coat in the dressing. Serve.

Makes: 1 portion / Prep time: 10 min
GLUTEN-FREE, VEGETARIAN

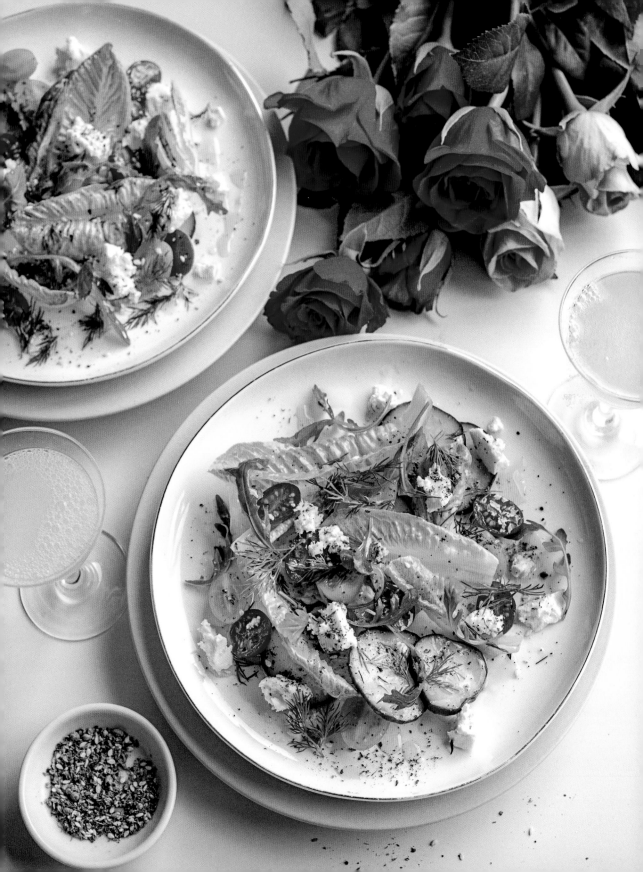

THE BEIGE BOWL

What you need:

1 x 7–ounce/200g jar of marinated artichoke hearts in oil, drained (about 5¾ ounces/160g drained weight)

2 tablespoons finely grated Parmesan

2 tablespoons toasted and chopped hazelnuts, blanched if you prefer

zest and juice of ½ unwaxed lemon

+ salt and pepper

Transport yourself into a monochromatic world where everything is a shade of beige, and devour this veggie starter. Oh, what's that? More Parmesan? Yes, indeed.

How to make it:

● Arrange the **artichokes** on a serving plate and sprinkle with the grated **Parmesan**, toasted and chopped **hazelnuts**, and the **lemon zest** and **juice**. Season well with **salt** and **pepper**, and serve.

Makes: 1 portion / Prep time: 5 min
GLUTEN-FREE, VEGETARIAN

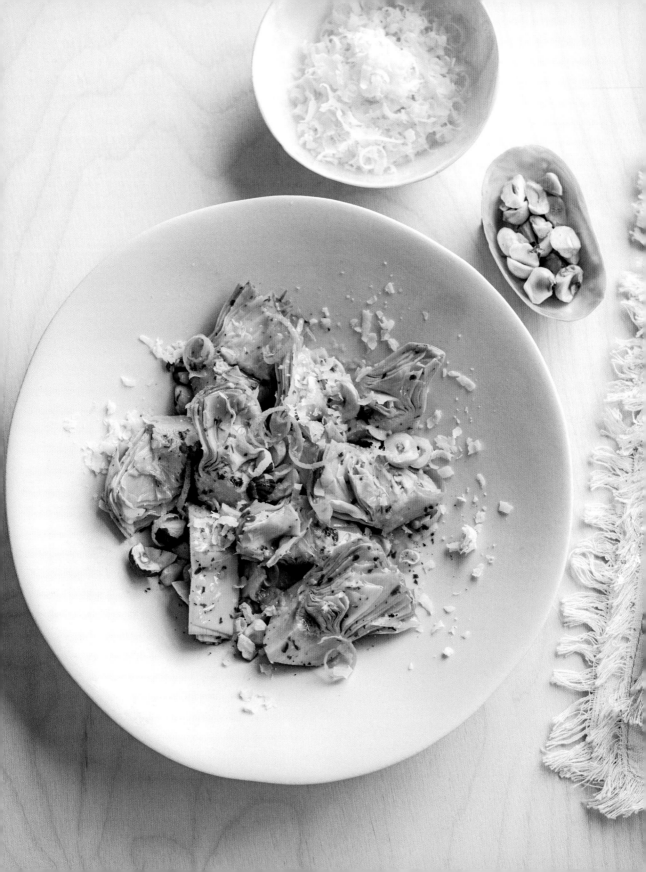

TALENTED TOMATOES

What you need:

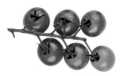

15 cherry tomatoes, halved

1 heaping tablespoon full-fat Greek yogurt

1 teaspoon dried oregano

+ **1 tablespoon olive oil**
+ **salt and pepper**

Tomatoes are not only a wonderful source of fiber for our veggie starter, they are also very good at holding on to that dreamy yogurt dressing so that it actually gets to our mouth. So much talent.

How to make it:

● In a bowl, place the **tomato** halves and add the **yogurt**, **oregano**, and **olive oil**. Stir everything together, then season generously with **salt** and **pepper**, and serve.

Makes: 1 portion / Prep time: 7 min
GLUTEN-FREE

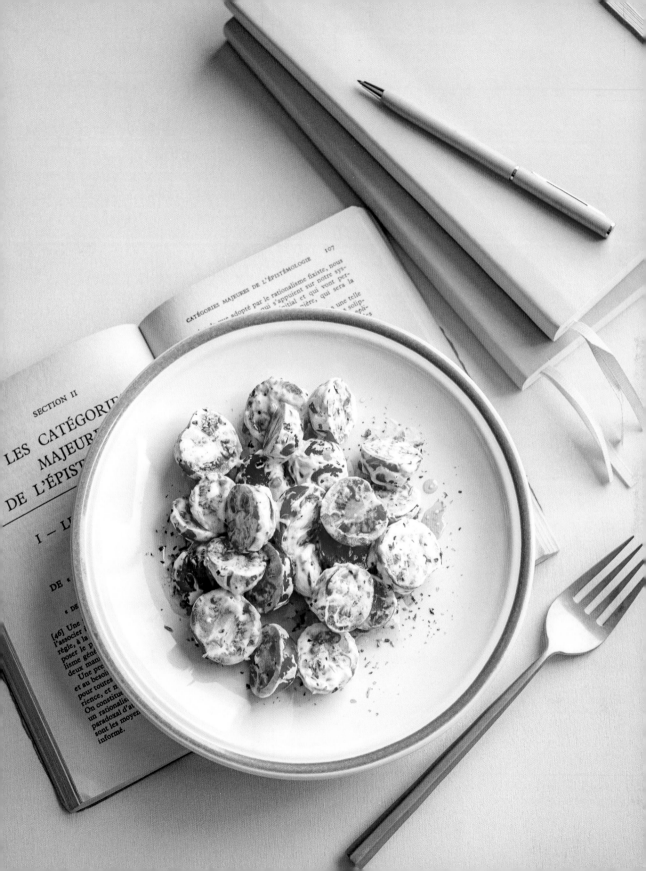

REMEMBERED HERB SALAD

What you need:

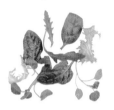

a small handful of mixed
lettuce leaves

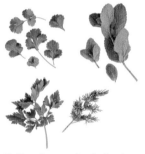

6–7 sprigs each of cilantro,
mint, parsley, and dill,
stemmed

juice of ½ lemon

+ 1 tablespoon olive oil
+ salt and pepper

"Hey, it's me. The herbs you bought and left in the back of your fridge. Do you remember me? I'd love to be in this tasty veggie starter and help your glucose be steady."

How to make it:

● Toss all the **lettuce leaves** and the **herb** leaves together in a bowl. Drizzle with the **lemon juice** and dress with the **olive oil**. Season with **salt** and **pepper**, and serve.

Makes: 1 portion / Prep time: 5 min
GLUTEN-FREE, VEGAN

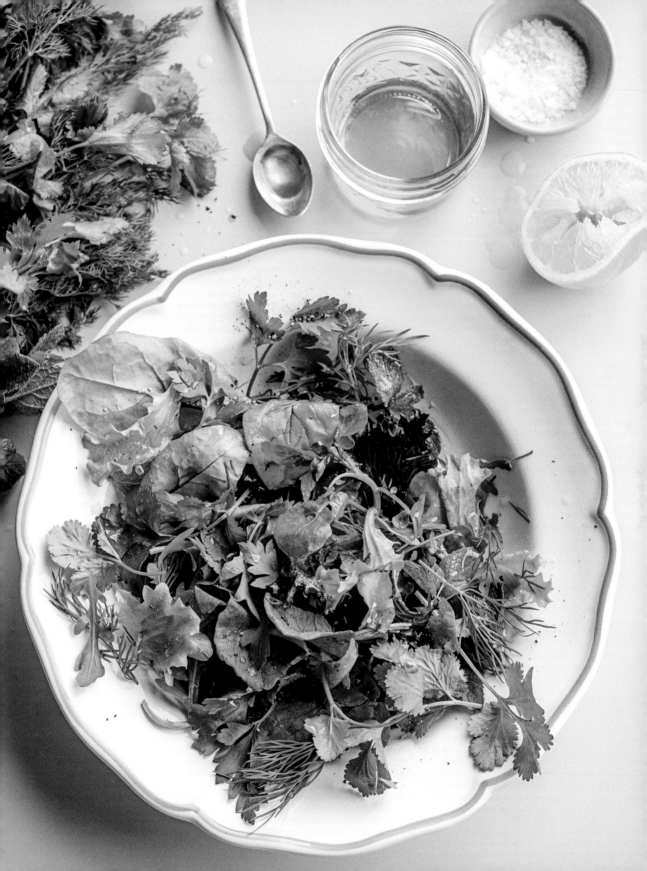

BEAUTIFUL BEETS

What you need:

3–4 cooked small baby beets, sliced

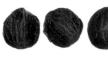

a small handful of dill, stems trimmed, leaves finely chopped

a small handful of hazelnuts, roughly chopped

+ 1 tablespoon olive oil
+ salt and pepper

Easy, breezy, beautiful. Beet.

How to make it:

● Combine the sliced **beets**, chopped **dill**, chopped **hazelnuts**, and **olive oil** in a bowl. Season with **salt** and **pepper**, and serve.

Makes: 1 portion / Prep time: 5 min
GLUTEN-FREE, VEGAN

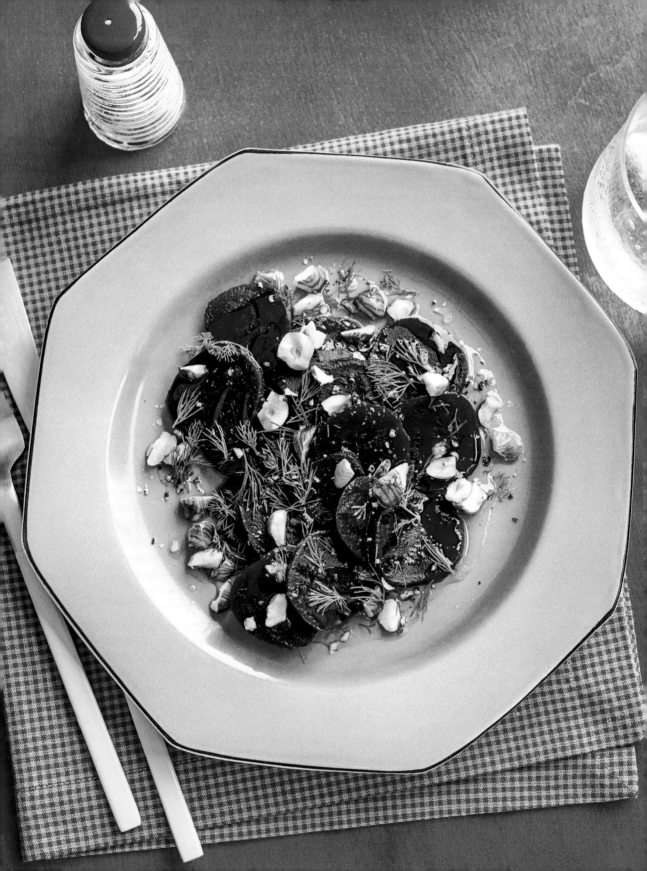

Tim Spector's
SQUISHY TOMATOES

What you need:

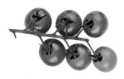

15 cherry tomatoes

1 large garlic clove, sliced

3–5 little gem or romaine heart lettuce leaves

+ 2 tablespoons olive oil
+ salt and pepper

Tim Spector is a glucose genius, and his squishy tomatoes recipe might just serve as the best evidence of that. Tim graciously allowed me to include his original creation here, and I am delighted to get to share it.

How to make it:

● Preheat the oven to 400°F. Place the **tomatoes**, sliced **garlic**, and **olive oil** in a small roasting dish (they need to have a snug fit) and season them with **salt** and **pepper**. Roast the tomatoes in the oven for 15 minutes, until they have collapsed and released their juices.

● Remove the dish from the oven and let the tomatoes cool slightly, then serve with leaves of **little gem** or **romaine**. Scoop up the succulent, juicy tomatoes with each little leaf!

Makes: 1 portion / Prep time: 3 min / Total cook time: 15 min
GLUTEN-FREE, VEGAN

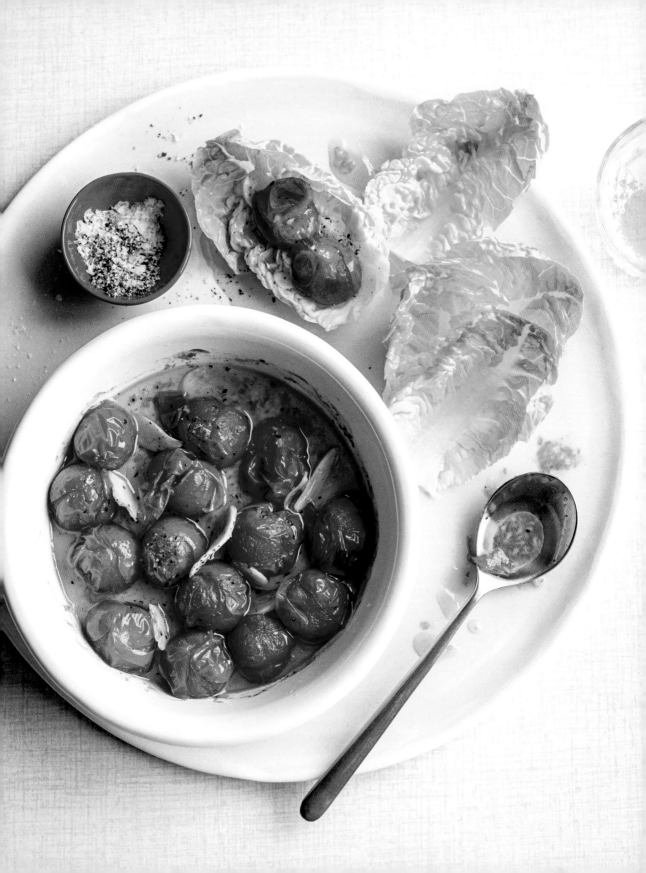

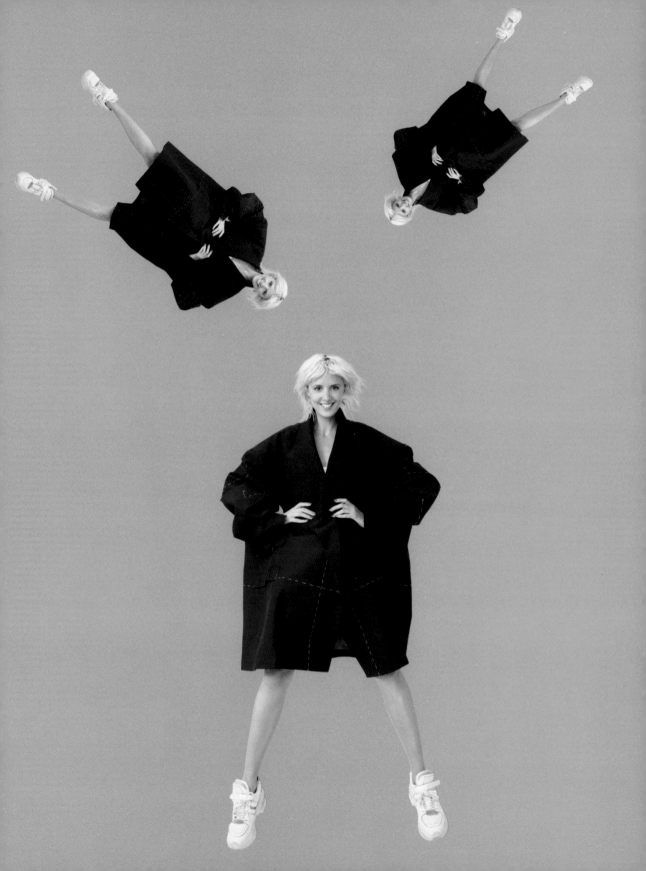

MOVEMENT

Your cells are making energy more efficiently, your brain is working better, your body is learning to burn fat for fuel, and your hormones are getting back on track. Bravo!

TESTIMONIALS FROM THE COMMUNITY

"I still can't believe all these little changes that you are hardly aware of but together they make a big change . . . and I don't want, I DON'T WANT, the Method to end. I am happy, calm, and serene."

"I'm in my forties and have had acne all my life. After one week on the Method, my skin started to improve; after four weeks it is almost clear. These are no longer hacks, they are my life!"

"When I started the movement, it changed everything. That's when I really started seeing results. It inspired me to kick everything up to 100 percent, and that's only made everything better. I'm so happy I did this."

"The best thing is that I don't have that constant feeling of hunger and I don't feel any anxiety anymore."

"My period is back!!"

"No migraines. I normally had two or three migraines a week and relied on daily medication. I had to come off the medication a few months ago and was really suffering without the meds. I was about to go back to them but thought I would give the program a go, as I had nothing to lose. Had a few headaches in the first few days, but haven't had any since! I am amazed with the results and so happy."

"With this program, it's as if I've finally become myself: I no longer have mood swings, and I greet bad news with a certain detachment. I always thought these problems were psychological and I did a lot of work on myself, but now I realize that it was purely physiological. I had tried diets (vegan, sugar-free, gluten-free, lactose-free), but what I like about this Method is that you can eat anything, there is no avoidance. The hacks are not difficult to integrate and I will follow them for the rest of my life (when it's easy, of course!)."

"Movement after meals definitely makes me happier. Even when I don't feel like going outside, I go for a walk and it changes everything."

"Sleep has improved, especially when I have been for a walk after dinner. I feel like it also calmed my mind down, which is a plus. The heat flashes I experience often after meals have improved—not gone away completely, but much better."

"I eat in a much more serene way, even if I decide to eat something for pleasure."

"Today when I was shopping, my choices were naturally much healthier. My desire was to buy some shrimp to make a ramen for the weekend. I laughed at this!"

"My workouts have changed: I feel more energetic, stronger, and more able to face hard exercises. Yesterday was my first day of unilateral hyperextensions and . . . achievement unlocked!"

"The biggest change for me is probably the steps I now take to prepare for a meal and then after a meal. I have my apple cider vinegar drink while I'm preparing, I eat my veggie starter first, and then I do a little bit of exercise after. Sometimes that's just cleaning the kitchen; sometimes it's playing with my dog; and sometimes it's doing a little dance. I've also had a shift in mentality in that if I don't do those things, I haven't failed. It's more a lifestyle of do them when it's practical and you can, and not to be hard on yourself if you miss a few."

"I do not have cravings anymore! In general I didn't have that many, but in the week before my period it was very obvious. No more cravings for me!"

"Life is so fun when you don't have food on your mind all the time! I can go food shopping without being tempted to buy something sweet, and I no longer notice my colleague eating a cookie. . . . This way it's really easy to just eat what your body needs."

"Although weight loss wasn't a goal for me, I think I've lost a few pounds anyway. Big bonus!"

"My life has totally changed, and my mental health has improved tremendously! I CAN'T THANK this Method enough. IT HAS CHANGED MY LIFE COMPLETELY!"

"I feel full of energy and less dependent on food!!! Yaaaaaaaaaaaay! No more ice cream at midnight!"

Your objective for Week 4

Wow. You are amazing. As we ride into the fourth and final week of the Method, just pause for a second and take in what you've done. You can be proud to have invested so much into your happiness and health.

I hope you've found that these hacks are slowly turning into habits for you, and are becoming tools that you will keep in your toolbox for life. Let's now meet the final tool of the Method—one that will recruit some very powerful glucose allies that cannot wait to be of help: your muscles.

Your objective during this last week is to continue with your savory breakfast, vinegar, and veggie starter hacks, and to layer in something that does not involve eating or drinking: movement.

After one meal per day, use your muscles for 10 minutes. Put simply, that means: ***move after eating.*** You should do this ideally within 90 minutes of the end of one of your meals, and the movement can be as simple as going for a 10-minute walk or doing calf raises at your desk, or as involved as corralling your colleagues and organizing an office dance party in the break room to your three favorite songs. What? It happens.

Some of you may already have some post-meal movement baked into your days (walking to work after breakfast, going on a coffee break after lunch, doing the dishes after dinner . . .), which means you are completing this objective every day without needing to be prompted. If so, great! Keep going. If not, there are lots of ideas for you in the next few pages.

No more recipes this week. Instead I'm going to showcase lots of ways in which you can get that movement in. And if 10 minutes feels like a lot, start with 1 minute and work your way up.

The science

There are multiple traditions that recommend walking after eating, such as the Indian custom of "100 steps after a meal," and they exist for good reason.

As I explained in the introduction to this book, our cells need glucose for energy. And the main way we provide glucose to our cells is by eating sweet and starchy foods, which contain glucose. The problem is that our modern diets tend to deliver too much glucose too quickly to our body—far more than it needs or can make use of. This creates glucose spikes.

Imagine, for example, you've just eaten a meal that leads to a glucose spike. As soon as this influx of glucose hits your body, two things can happen. If you stay sedentary as the spike reaches its peak, extra glucose will flood your cells and overwhelm your mitochondria. This increases inflammation and causes the excess glucose to be stored away in the liver, muscles, and fat.

On the other hand, **if you move after eating, some of the glucose you have just eaten gets used up by your muscle cells**. Your mitochondria turn the extra glucose into energy to fuel your contracting muscles, and the spike reduces. On a continuous glucose monitor graph, the difference is stark.

And here's the kicker: when we move after eating, we flatten our glucose curve *without increasing our insulin level*—just as we do when we drink vinegar. Although our muscles usually need insulin to stash glucose away, they don't when they are in the act of contracting. They don't need insulin to take up glucose. This is excellent news, as reducing our insulin levels is a key factor that improves our health—too much insulin in the body being the driver of many conditions, such as polycystic ovary syndrome and type 2 diabetes.

All in all, moving for 10 minutes after a meal is a very powerful hack to flatten our glucose curves, and the joy is that it doesn't require us to change anything about what we are eating. Also, if you sometimes experience a "food coma" after eating, this hack will nip that right in the bud.

How using our muscles can reduce a glucose spike

How to make your own movement hack

After a meal or after a snack, move your body in any way that is easy, as long as you aren't still and some of your muscles are activating. It is really up to you. Maybe it's stretching or ice-skating, maybe it's painting your walls, maybe it's shopping, maybe it's having sex (yes, that counts, too!).

How to know if you're doing it right

You are doing it right if you can find a movement that easily fits into your life and that feels like a treat. As I've said, you may already be doing something that counts for this hack. You should also feel good after doing it, not in pain or out of breath or exhausted. We're talking light movement here, during which you can take some time for yourself, have a break from work, listen to some music, have fun, call a friend, or get something done around the house that you wanted to do anyway. Don't try to shoehorn complicated or exhausting movement into your schedule.

   Take a moment to review your daily activities to see if you're already completing this hack: Are there times during the day when you walk somewhere? Does your job require you to be active and not sitting down? Do you tidy your home, walk your dog, or grocery shop? If you can time these activities to happen within 90 minutes of the end of a meal, you'll be checking off this hack. See pages 224–25 for more examples of the movement hack.

Tips from the community

• Transform a phone call into a walking phone call. While on the phone, get up and walk around—your home, your office, the block. You'll get your hack in.

• A very popular technique is the 10-minute walk after lunch.

• Tidying your kitchen or your place after eating is a great way to complete this hack.

- If you don't feel like getting up right after eating (that's understandable, and you don't need to), set a timer on your phone for 80 minutes to remind you to do some movement then, at the very end of the spike-slashing window.

- Use the seated calf raises movement (page 225) at your desk while you are sitting down at work.

- Keep a weight or heavy object by your couch, and if you watch TV after dinner, do some bicep curls with it.

Common questions from the community

What if I'm at the office and there is nowhere to walk? At the office, the easiest ways to complete the hack are: go up and down some stairs a few times (if your office is in a building with stairs), or do calf raises at your desk (while sitting down, push onto your toes and raise your heels up and down under your desk for 10 minutes—more information on how to do this on page 225).

Does it have to be within 90 minutes after the end of the meal? Yes!

After which meal is it best to complete this hack? The best time to complete this hack is when it is easiest for you to do it.

Can I do the movement before eating? You can move anytime you want, but to complete this hack, the movement needs to be within a 90-minute window *after* eating.

Can I do the movement at the same time as I eat? Yes, that works. But some people find it uncomfortable to move while eating, so it's a less popular choice.

Can I have my main course, then move while eating dessert? Yes!

Can it be after breakfast? Yes. After any meal. (Or after a snack.)

I go to the gym in the morning before breakfast— I'm already exercising a lot every day. Do I still need to do this hack? Ideally, yes: if you can find 10 minutes for some extra movement *after* one of your meals every day, your glucose will thank you.

Do I need to do this hack even if my meals aren't high in glucose? Yes. While moving after eating is most useful to curb a glucose spike from a meal that contains starches or sugars, even if your meal does not contain starches or sugars, it is still helpful to your body. Test it out and make it a habit.

I cannot easily move. What should I do? Feel free to skip this hack, and continue on with the savory breakfast, vinegar, and veggie starter. You're already doing amazingly!

LIST OF IDEAS TO COMPLETE THE MOVEMENT HACK

- Stretch

- Walk while listening to a podcast

- Go outside and stroll around for a bit—breathe in the fresh air

- Walk to or from somewhere or walk your dog

- Walk on a treadmill

- Do a 10-minute YouTube dance video

- Put on your three favorite songs and dance on your own

- Do the dishes

- Clean your kitchen or home

- Tidy

- Vacuum

- Repair something

- Go up and down stairs

- If your job requires you to be on your feet, just continue doing that

- Run an errand

- Go grocery shopping

- Do seated calf raises: While sitting down and with both feet on the floor, holding on to the table with your hands, press through the balls of your feet to raise your heels, set them back down, and repeat. Do this for 10 minutes. This activates your soleus muscle, which is a calf muscle that is particularly helpful in soaking up glucose from the blood.

- Play with your kids

- Do some squats while watching TV

- Do jump squats

- Lift some heavy objects (weights or water bottles) while watching TV

- Go to a Pilates class or any other type of class

- Go for a hike

- Bike

- Go to the gym

- Do any kind of exercise

- Play a team sport

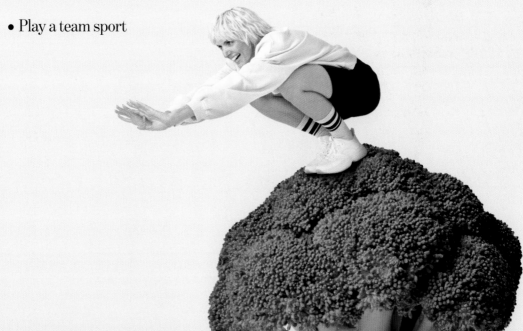

ANYTIME MAIN DISHES

Want some glucose-steadying recipes for lunch and dinner, or after your veggie starter? You're in the right place. Come on in.

ROASTED RED PEPPER *and* FENNEL *with* CAPERS, LE PUY LENTILS, *and* CHICKEN

What you need:

2 red bell peppers, seeded and cut into quarters

1 fennel bulb, cut into thin wedges (reserve the fronds if you have any)

2 skin-on, bone-in chicken thighs

1 tablespoon capers, drained

1⅔ cups/125g cooked Le Puy lentils

a small bunch of flat-leaf parsley, roughly chopped, to serve (optional)

+ 2 tablespoons olive oil
+ salt and pepper

Long live the sheet pan dish! Anytime I can reduce my washing up, I'm in. This sheet pan dish is as pretty on the plate as it is pleasing for the palate.

How to make it:

● Preheat the oven to 400°F. Arrange the quartered **red bell peppers**, wedges of **fennel**, and **chicken thighs** on a sheet pan, drizzle them with the **olive oil**, and season with **salt** and **pepper**. Roast the vegetables and chicken in the oven for 30 minutes, until the vegetables are softened and charred a little, and the chicken is cooked through.

● Remove the sheet pan from the oven and scatter the drained **capers** and cooked **Le Puy lentils** all over the chicken and vegetables. Return the sheet pan to the oven for 5 minutes more, until the lentils are heated through. Serve topped with the parsley and fennel fronds, if using.

Makes: 2 portions / Prep time: 10 min / Total cook time: 35 min
GLUTEN-FREE

MY FAVORITE SAN FRANCISCO SALAD

COUNTS AS YOUR VINEGAR HACK FOR THE DAY AS WELL

What you need:

½ red onion, thinly sliced

2 tablespoons apple cider vinegar

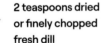

2 skinless, boneless chicken breasts (about 5¾ ounces/ 160g each), sliced in half horizontally through their middle (to make them thinner)

3 tablespoons full-fat Greek yogurt

2 teaspoons dried or finely chopped fresh dill

1 grapefruit, peeled and gently squeezed to release 1 tablespoon of juice, before being cut into segments, juice reserved

3½ ounces/100g kale, tough stalks removed, leaves sliced

1 head of little gem lettuce or romaine heart, leaves separated

+ 4 tablespoons/60ml olive oil

+ salt and pepper

When I like something, I stick with it. When I was living in San Francisco, I fell in love with a salad just like this one from a Greek restaurant. I probably had it twice a week for four years! So here is my take on it. I hope you'll love it as much as I do.

How to make it:

● In a bowl, place the sliced **red onion** and cover it with the **apple cider vinegar**. Mix them together well and set aside to pickle while you make the chicken.

● Heat 2 tablespoons of the **olive oil** in a large frying pan on high heat. Season the thin **chicken pieces** with **salt** and **pepper** and add them to the pan. Fry them for 3 minutes on each side, or until they are cooked through, then remove them from the pan, cut them into thin slices, and set them aside.

● In a large bowl, mix the **yogurt**, **dill**, **grapefruit juice**, and the remaining **olive oil** and season it generously with salt and pepper to make a dressing.

● Add the sliced **kale** to the bowl and massage it with your hands for a few minutes, until the kale is softened and thoroughly coated with the dressing.

● Add the **little gem or romaine** leaves and toss them in the dressing with the kale.

● Divide the dressed leaves between two bowls and top each portion with the **grapefruit segments**, pickled red onion, and sliced chicken, then serve.

Makes: 2 portions / Prep time: 10 min / Total cook time: 7 min
GLUTEN-FREE

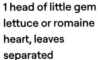

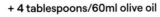

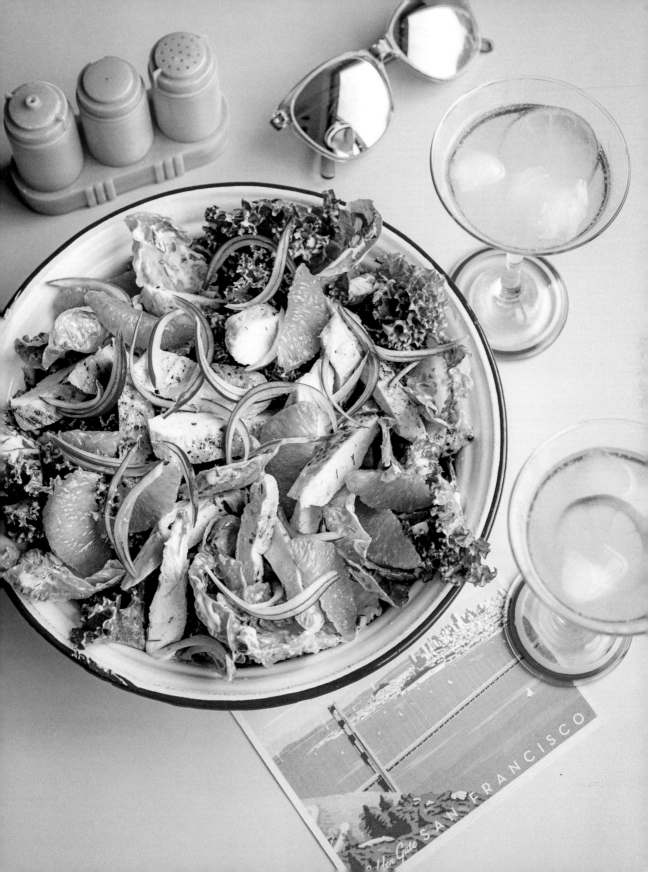

TAHINI BAKED COD

What you need:

2 skinless, boneless cod fillets

2 shallots, finely chopped

3 tablespoons tahini

⅓ cup/80ml boiling water plus extra if needed

a generous handful of dill, stemmed, leaves finely chopped

zest and juice of ½ unwaxed lemon

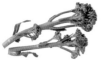

12¼ ounces/350g Broccolini, tough ends trimmed

+ 2 tablespoons olive oil
+ salt and pepper

What's a person to do when the craving for a deeply rich and creamy meal strikes, but the desire to keep their glucose steady strikes even harder? Well, whip up this recipe, of course. I adore it, and I hope you will, too.

How to make it:

● Preheat the oven to 425°F and line a sheet pan with parchment paper. Place the **cod fillets** on the lined sheet pan and drizzle them with 1 tablespoon of the **olive oil** and season with **salt** and **pepper**. Roast the fillets in the oven for 10–12 minutes, until cooked through.

● Meanwhile, make the sauce. Heat the remaining **olive oil** in a medium frying pan on medium heat. Add the chopped **shallots**. Fry them for about 5 minutes, or until they are softened.

● Add the **tahini** and **boiling water** and stir the sauce on low heat for about 3 minutes, until it's nice and smooth, like the consistency of heavy cream. Add more boiling water if necessary.

● Stir in the chopped **dill** leaves and the **lemon zest** and **juice**, and season with salt and pepper.

● Steam or blanch the **Broccolini** for 4–5 minutes, until tender. Serve it with the cod and tahini sauce.

Makes: 2 portions / Prep time: 5 min / Total cook time: 12 min

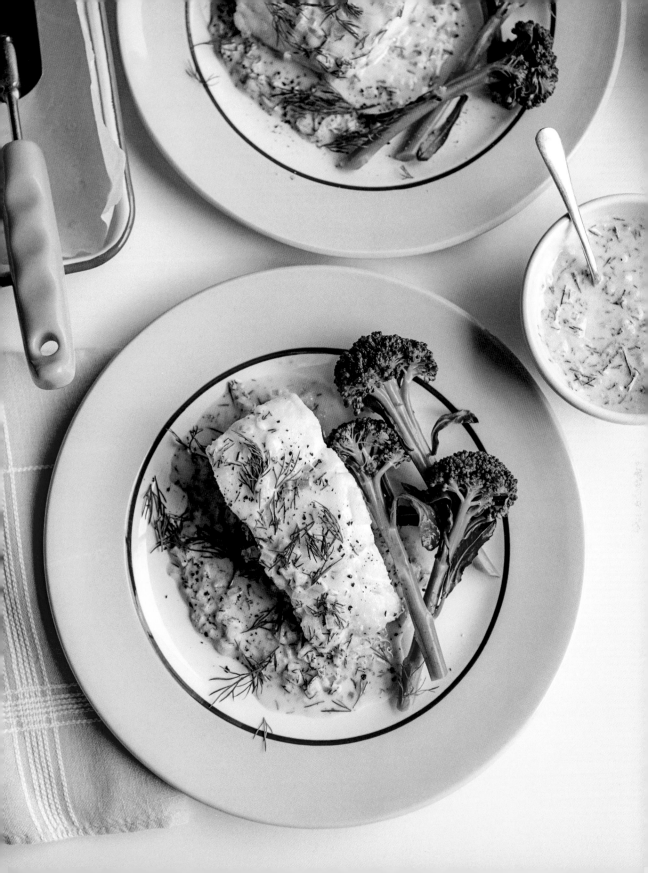

GROWN-UP TUNA PITA

What you need:

1 x 5-ounce/140g can of tuna in oil, drained

1 tablespoon Dijon mustard

1 tablespoon mayonnaise

1 heaping teaspoon capers, drained

1 pita bread

2–3 iceberg, romaine, or little gem lettuce leaves

+ salt and pepper

Ahhh, the classic tuna sandwich. This is a version I learned from a dear friend. The capers and mustard add a zingy element to the original, making it the perfect elevated version of a middle school staple.

How to make it:

- In a bowl, mix the **tuna**, **Dijon mustard**, **mayonnaise**, and **capers** together and season them with **salt** and **pepper**.

- Toast the **pita bread** and open it up to create a pocket. Stuff the toasted pita with the **lettuce leaves** and the tuna filling, and serve.

Makes: 1 portion / Prep time: 10 min

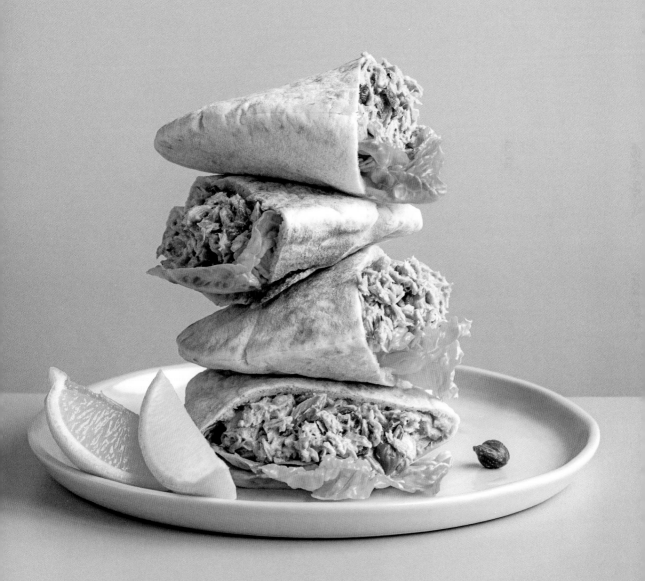

MASON JAR

What you need:

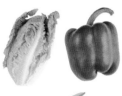
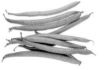

a handful of mixed salad veggies, such as lettuce, bell peppers, green onions, and green beans, chopped into bite-size pieces

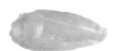

1 cooked chicken breast, sliced

2–3 tablespoons cooked white or brown rice

a dressing of your choice

This recipe has endless possibilities once you follow the basic principle (veggies on the bottom, protein in the middle, starch on the top). Pack it, take it to work, flip it on a plate . . . And there you are—your food more or less set up to be eaten in the right order: veggies first and carbs last. Don't fret if you don't eat everything exactly in that order; a general intention is what matters.

Use any veg and leaves you have in your fridge. Protein could be chicken, beef, hard-boiled eggs, tofu . . . and then you could add some cooked rice or pasta. Simple additions like pesto, harissa, or even mayo will make a perfect topping, or turn to pages 136–39 for some inspiration for dressings that also pack a vinegar hack.

How to make it:

● Build your mason jar. Start with a layer of the **salad veggies**, then follow with the **chicken** slices, and top with the cooked **rice**.

● To serve, tip all the contents of the jar out onto a plate, pour the **dressing** over the top, and enjoy!

Makes: 1 portion / Prep time: 10 min
GLUTEN-FREE

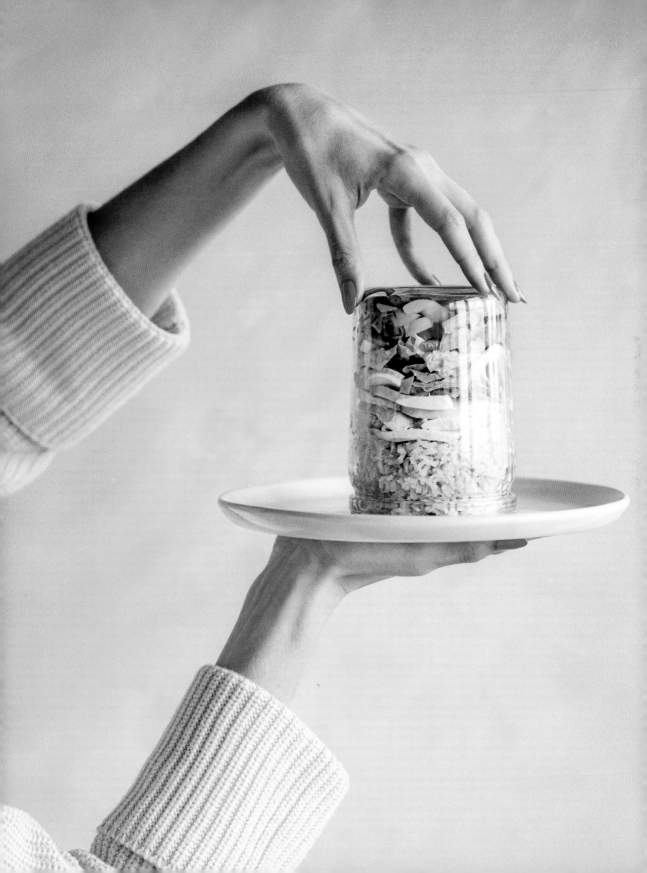

Jessie's NIÇOISE SALAD

What you need:

2 eggs

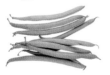

3½ ounces/100g green beans, trimmed

1½ tablespoons Dijon mustard

juice of 1 lemon

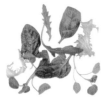

2 large handfuls of mixed lettuce leaves

2 x 5-ounce/140g cans of tuna in olive oil, drained

+ 2 tablespoons olive oil
+ salt and pepper

I don't want to brag but . . . okay, yes I do! I make a mean niçoise salad. And because I like you, I'm going to share my top-secret, never-before-revealed recipe with you . . . just keep it between us, okay?

How to make it:

● Bring a small saucepan of water to a boil on high heat. Add the **eggs** and boil them for 5 minutes, then add the **green beans**. Boil for 2 minutes more, until the beans are just cooked and the eggs are gooey-hard boiled. Drain everything in a colander.

● Remove the beans from the colander and set them aside. Then run the eggs under cold water to prevent them from cooking further. When the eggs are cool enough to handle, peel them and set them aside.

● Make the dressing. In a bowl, whisk the **Dijon mustard**, **lemon juice**, and **olive oil** together, and season with **salt** and **pepper**. Whisk until the dressing ingredients have emulsified.

● In a large bowl, toss the **lettuce leaves** with half the dressing and divide them between two serving bowls or plates. Top each portion with equal amounts of the **tuna** and green beans.

● Cut each egg in half and place the egg halves on top of each salad portion. Season with salt and pepper once more, and drizzle the remaining dressing over all. Serve.

Makes: 2 portions / Prep time: 12 min / Total cook time: 7 min
GLUTEN-FREE

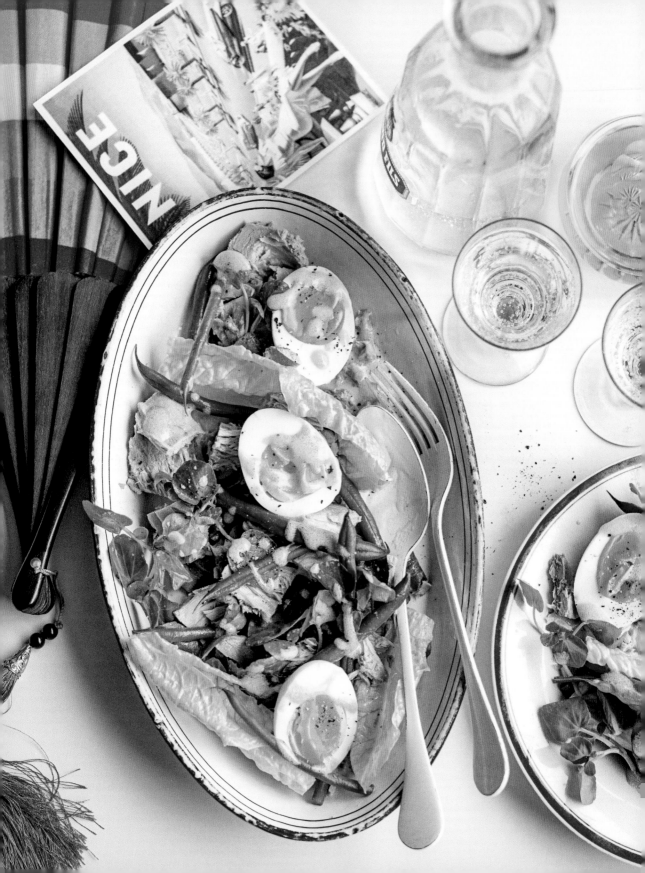

CHILE GARLIC SHRIMP

What you need:

3 garlic cloves, roughly chopped

1 red chile, roughly chopped

½ lemon, cut into small wedges

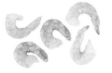

1 pound/450g shelled raw large shrimp

a big handful of flat-leaf parsley, stemmed, leaves roughly chopped steamed green

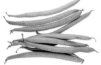

beans and crusty bread, to serve (optional)

+ 3 tablespoons olive oil
+ salt and pepper

Warning: While this main dish is absolutely exquisite, the chile + garlic combo might not be one you want to indulge in before a date. The flavors are strong, and so is their ability to stick to your lips.

How to make it:

● Heat the **olive oil** in a large frying pan on medium heat. Add the chopped **garlic** and chopped **red chile** and fry them for 1½ minutes, to soften.

● Add the **lemon** wedges and **shrimp** and cook them for about 3 minutes, stirring all the time, until the shrimp have turned pink and are cooked through. Season with **salt** and **pepper**, and stir in the chopped **parsley.**

● Serve with some steamed green beans and maybe some crusty bread to mop up the juices, if you like.

Makes: 2 portions / Prep time: 5 min / Total cook time: 5 min
GLUTEN-FREE

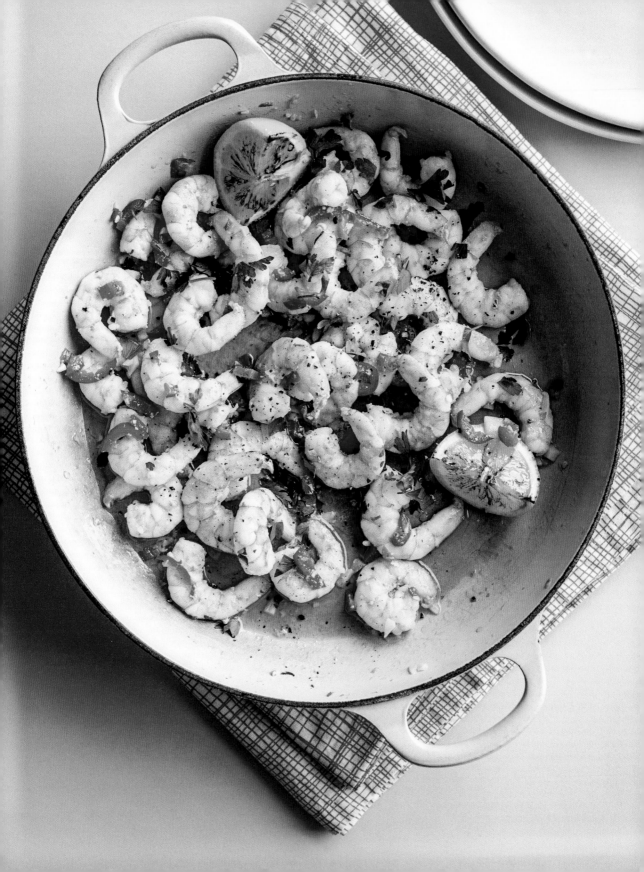

CHICKPEA PEPERONATA
with RIB-EYE STEAK

COUNTS AS YOUR VINEGAR HACK FOR THE DAY AS WELL

What you need:

 1 small onion, sliced

 2 red or yellow bell peppers, seeded and thinly sliced

 3–4 thyme sprigs, stemmed

 2 garlic cloves, sliced

 1 x 15-ounce/ 425g can of chickpeas, drained

 2 tablespoons balsamic vinegar

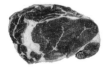

2 rib-eye steaks (7 ounces/ 200g each)

+ 2½ tablespoons olive oil
+ salt and pepper

When the mood strikes for a particularly satisfying, filling meal . . . right this way!

How to make it:

● Make the peperonata. Heat 1½ tablespoons of the **olive oil** in a saucepan on medium heat. Add the sliced **onion**, sliced **bell peppers**, and the **thyme** leaves and fry for 10 minutes, stirring from time to time, until the vegetables have softened.

● Add the sliced **garlic**, **chickpeas**, and **balsamic vinegar** and cook, covered, for 3–4 minutes more, until the garlic has softened and the vinegar has reduced a little.

● Meanwhile, place a griddle pan on high heat. Season the **rib-eye steaks** with **salt** and **pepper** and brush the remaining olive oil all over them. When the pan is smoking hot, grill the steaks for 2–3 minutes on each side (for medium-rare). When the steaks are done, remove them from the heat, cover them with foil, and let them rest for 5 minutes.

● When you're ready to serve, season the peperonata with salt and pepper, slice the steak thinly, and divide everything between two plates to serve.

Makes: 2 portions / Prep time: 10 min / Total cook time: 15 min
GLUTEN-FREE

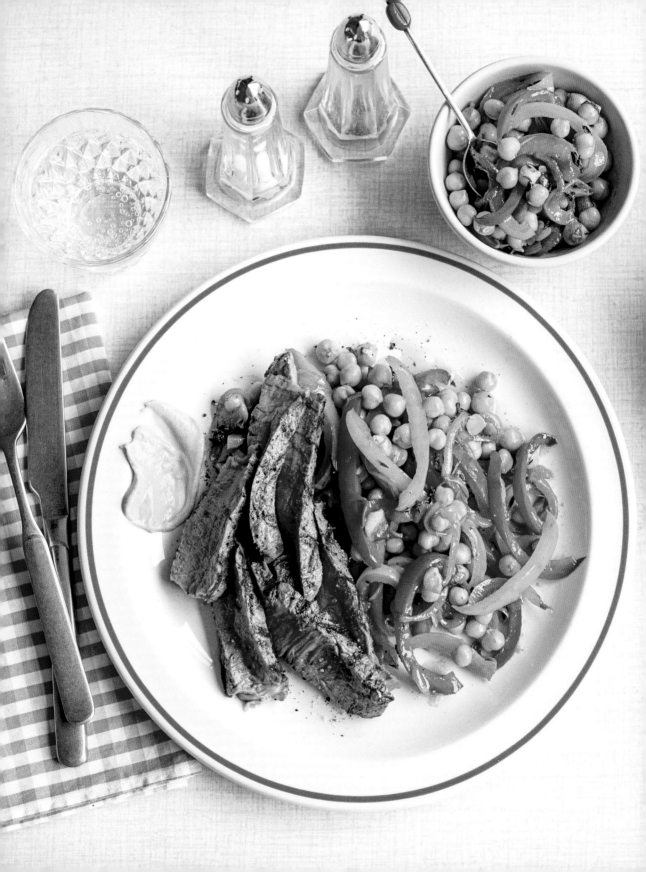

STEAMED SILKEN TOFU *with a* CHILE, GARLIC, *and* GINGER SAUCE

What you need:

1 x 10½-ounce/ 300g block of silken tofu, halved

1 head of bok choy, sliced lengthwise into quarters

2-inch/5cm piece of ginger, peeled and finely chopped

2 garlic cloves, sliced

2 tablespoons soy sauce (or tamari, if you're gluten-free)

juice of ½ lime

½ teaspoon chile powder (as hot as you like)

any kind of cooked rice, to serve

+ 2 tablespoons olive oil

Chile, garlic, and ginger—as the great Julie Andrews once sang, "These are a few of my favorite things!" The flavorful sauce from this dish brings the tofu to life, and makes for a mouthwatering meal.

How to make it:

● If you have a bamboo steamer, use it. Otherwise, use a colander, a saucepan, and a small plate. For the latter method, pour 1 cup/ 240ml of **water** into a saucepan and suspend the colander on top—make sure you choose a saucepan that enables the colander to sit above the water level. Place the halved **tofu** on a small plate that fits inside the colander and carefully position it. Place the sliced **bok choy** alongside the tofu. Cover the colander tightly with a saucepan lid or another plate and steam the tofu and bok choy for 10 minutes, until the bok choy is tender.

● Meanwhile, heat the **olive oil** in a frying pan on medium heat. Add the chopped **ginger** and sliced **garlic**, then fry, stirring, for about 2 minutes, until the garlic is starting to turn golden.

● Add the **soy sauce or tamari** and **lime juice** and simmer for about 10 seconds, then remove the frying pan from the heat and stir in the **chile powder**.

● To serve, divide the tofu equally between two plates, divide out the bok choy, and top with the sauce. The dish goes well with any kind of cooked **rice**.

Makes: 2 portions / Prep time: 10 min / Total cook time: 12 min
GLUTEN-FREE (if using tamari), VEGAN

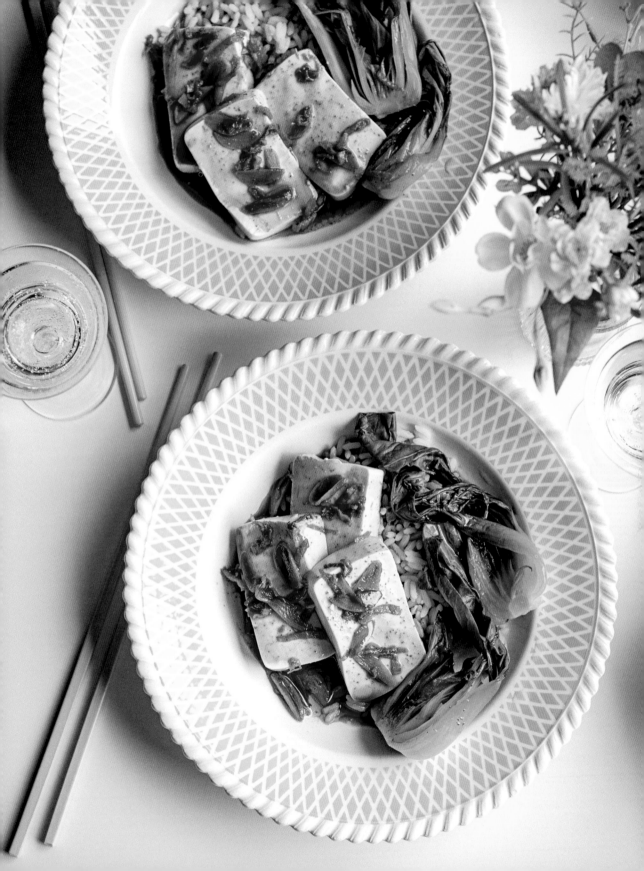

BAKED SALMON *with* CUCUMBER *and* PICKLED GINGER DRESSING

What you need:

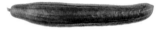

2 skinless, boneless salmon fillets (about 5¼ ounces/ 150g each)

3 tablespoons pickled ginger, drained and roughly chopped

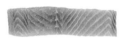

¼ cucumber, seeded and finely diced

a small bunch of cilantro, stemmed, leaves finely chopped

1 cup/200g cooked white or brown rice

2 teaspoons soy sauce (or tamari, if you're gluten-free; optional)

+ 1 tablespoon olive oil
+ salt and pepper

The flavors of this dish are subtle but craveable. Pickled ginger is available from most major supermarkets—if you haven't had any yet, run, don't walk!

How to make it:

● Preheat the oven to 400°F and line a roasting pan with parchment paper. Lay the **salmon fillets** on top, drizzle them with the **olive oil**, season them with **salt** and **pepper**, and bake them in the oven for 12 minutes, until the fillets are opaque and cooked through.

● Meanwhile, in a bowl, mix the chopped **pickled ginger**, diced **cucumber**, and chopped **cilantro** together and season the mixture with a little salt and pepper.

● When the salmon is ready, serve each fillet on a bed of cooked **rice** and piled high with the pickled ginger dressing. A drizzle of soy sauce or tamari is a lovely addition, but the dish is also lovely without.

Makes: 2 portions / Prep time: 10 min / Total cook time: 12 min
GLUTEN-FREE (if using tamari)

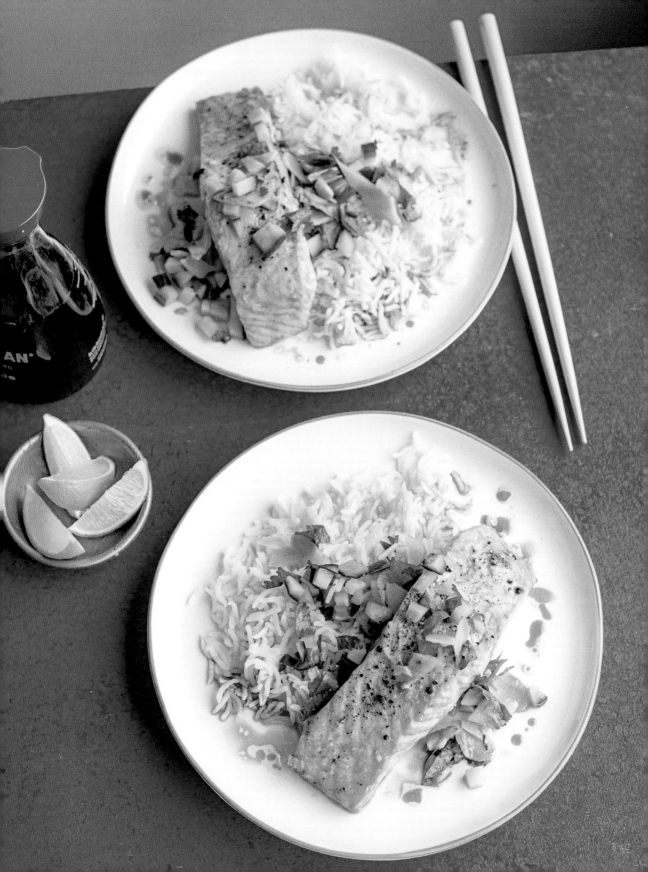

CHICKEN, LEMON, *and* OLIVE DISH

What you need:

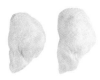

2 skin-on, bone-in chicken thighs

1 lemon, cut into wedges and seeds removed

¾ cup/100g pitted mixed olives

1 red chile, roughly chopped (optional)

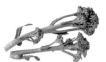

3½ ounces/100g Broccolini, tough ends trimmed

+ 2 tablespoons olive oil
+ salt and pepper

There are some meals that are so simple, classic, and tasty, they deserve a spot on every weekly glucose-steady meal lineup.

How to make it:

● Preheat the oven to 400°F. Place the **chicken thighs**, **lemon** wedges, **olives**, and chopped **red chile** (if using) in a roasting dish. Drizzle the **olive oil** over the top and season everything with **salt** and **pepper**, then roast it in the oven for 30 minutes, until the chicken thighs are cooked through.

● Remove the roasting dish from the oven and add the **Broccolini**. Return it all to the oven and roast for 5 minutes more, until the Broccolini is softened and charred a little. Divide the chicken and Broccolini between two serving plates, and serve.

Makes: 2 portions / Prep time: 7 min / Total cook time: 35 min
GLUTEN-FREE

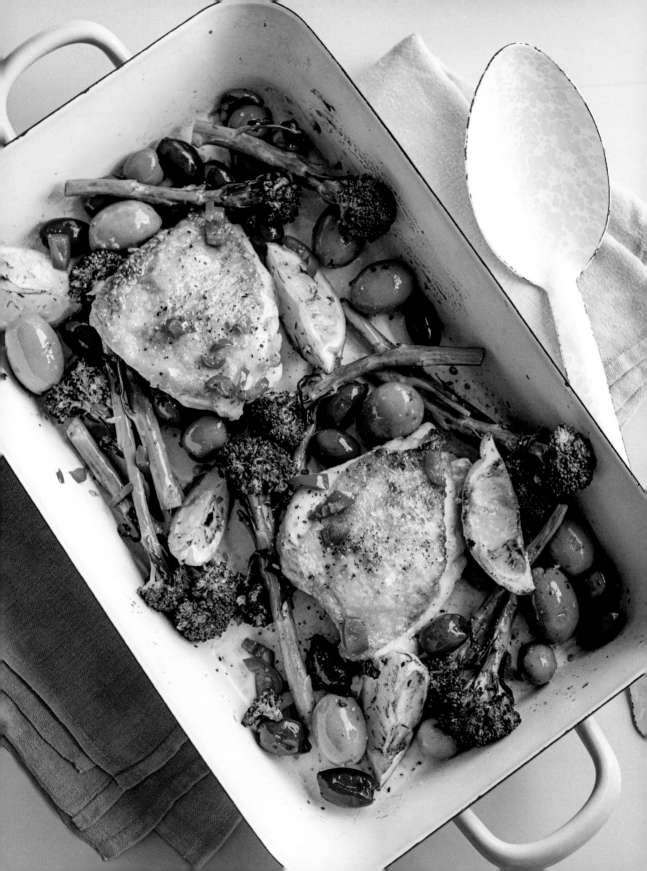

POACHED CHICKEN *with* GREEN ONION *and* GINGER

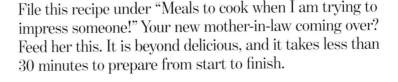

What you need:

2-inch/5cm piece of ginger, peeled

6 green onions

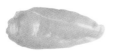

2 skinless, boneless chicken breasts (about 5¾ ounces/160g each)

1 garlic clove, chopped

2 tablespoons soy sauce (or tamari, if you're gluten-free)

1 cup/200g cooked quinoa or white or brown rice

+ 3 tablespoons olive oil

File this recipe under "Meals to cook when I am trying to impress someone!" Your new mother-in-law coming over? Feed her this. It is beyond delicious, and it takes less than 30 minutes to prepare from start to finish.

How to make it:

● Carefully cut 3 thin slices from the length of the **ginger** and finely chop the remainder. Leave 1 **green onion** whole, then finely slice the remaining 5 green onions, keeping the white and green parts separated.

● Place the **chicken breasts**, the whole green onion, and the 3 slices of ginger in a medium saucepan and cover them with water. Place the pan on high heat and bring the water to a boil. Then lower the heat and simmer for 15 minutes, until the chicken is cooked through. Set aside, leaving the chicken in the poaching liquid.

● Heat the **olive oil** in a frying pan on medium heat. Add the white parts of the chopped green onions and the chopped **garlic**, and fry them for a couple of minutes, until everything is starting to crisp and brown.

● Add the **soy sauce or tamari**, ½ cup/120ml of the chicken poaching liquid, the chopped ginger, and the green parts of the chopped green onions. Cook, stirring, for 1 minute, so that the sauce reduces a little and the ginger softens.

● Using a slotted spoon, remove the chicken from the remaining poaching liquid and cut it into thin slices.

● Divide the cooked **quinoa or rice** between two serving plates, then top each portion with the chicken slices. Pour the sauce over the top to finish, and serve.

Makes: 2 portions / Prep time: 7 min / Total cook time: 20 min
GLUTEN-FREE (if using tamari)

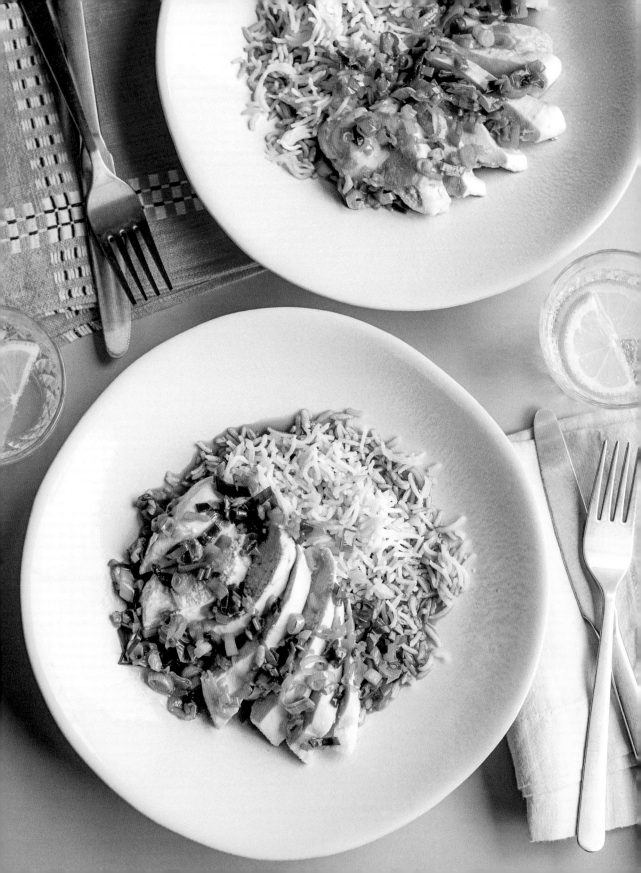

CRISPY BEEF BOWL
with kimchi

What you need:

7 ounces/200g ground beef (5% fat is good)

2 tablespoons sriracha

2 tablespoons soy sauce (or tamari, if you're gluten-free)

4 iceberg lettuce leaves, finely shredded

2 generous tablespoons kimchi

1 avocado, pitted and sliced

+ 2 tablespoons olive oil

For nights when all you want to do is curl up with some yummy food and relax. The sriracha adds a kick without being over-the-top spicy, and the avocado adds a cool, creamy texture. Absolutely divine!

How to make it:

● Heat the **olive oil** in a medium nonstick frying pan on medium heat. Add the **ground beef** and fry it for about 10 minutes, breaking it up with a wooden spoon, until it's browned all over and starting to become crispy. Stir in 1 tablespoon of the **sriracha** and all the **soy sauce or tamari**.

● Divide the shredded **iceberg lettuce** between two bowls, along with the **kimchi** and sliced **avocado**. Top with the crispy beef and drizzle the remaining sriracha on top.

Makes: 2 portions / Prep time: 10 min / Total cook time: 10 min
GLUTEN-FREE (if using tamari)

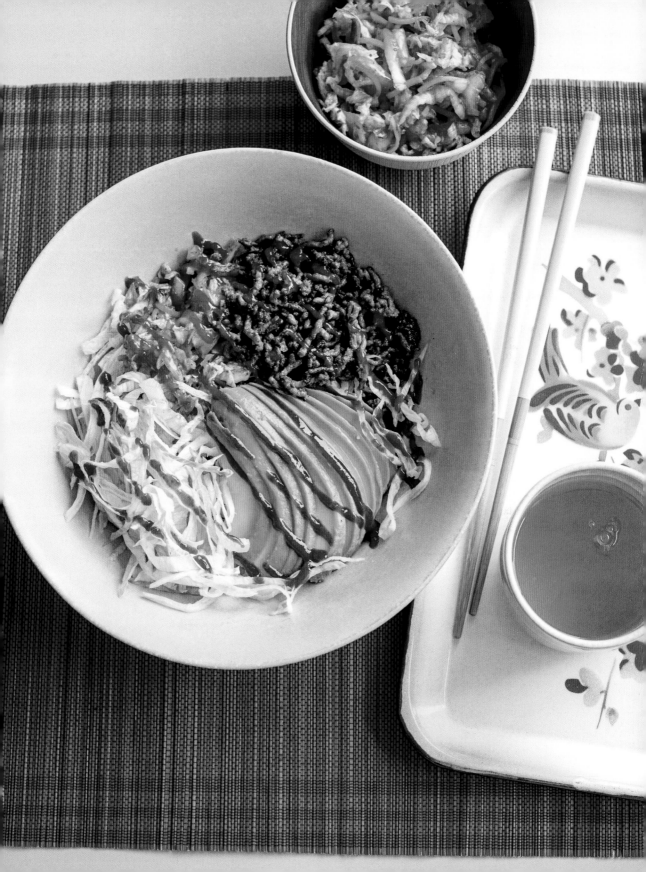

ANYTIME DESSERTS

I've said it before and I will say it again:
"Yes. I. Eat. Dessert!"
It's absolutely possible to eat sugar
and keep our glucose steady—we just
need to eat it after a meal, instead
of for breakfast or as a snack.

TOFFEE PEACH PAVLOVA

What you need:

½ cup/90g granulated sugar

⅓ cup/60g light-brown sugar

3 large egg whites

1 teaspoon white wine vinegar

7 tablespoons/100ml heavy cream, whipped; or 6 tablespoons/100g full-fat Greek yogurt

3 ripe peaches, pits removed, sliced; or ¾ cup/100g raspberries

+ a pinch of salt

The addition of light-brown sugar to a traditional meringue recipe creates the most intoxicating caramel toffee flavor. This is THE BEST! In terms of what fruit to use, peaches work particularly well, but choose what's in season and you won't go wrong.

How to make it:

● Preheat the oven to 350°F and line a baking sheet with parchment paper. In a bowl, mix the **granulated sugar** and **light-brown sugar** together so that there are no lumps.

● Place the **egg whites** and pinch of **salt** into the bowl of a stand mixer and whisk on high speed until the egg whites are stiff.

● A spoonful at a time, add the sugar mixture to the egg whites, whisking to incorporate between each addition.

● When you have added all the sugar, let the mixer run on high speed for 6 minutes, until you have a stiff and glossy meringue. Add the **white wine vinegar** and whisk for 1 minute more.

● Transfer the mixture to the prepared baking sheet, flattening it down to create a circle that is about 7 inches/18cm in diameter and 2 inches/5cm thick.

● Place the meringue base in the oven and immediately lower the heat to 275°F. Bake the meringue for 1½ hours, until it is crisp on the outside. Remove it from the oven and let cool. When you're ready to serve the pavlova, top it with the **whipped cream** or **Greek yogurt** and the sliced **peaches** or the **raspberries**.

Makes: 6 portions / Prep time: 15 min / Total cook time: 1½ hours
GLUTEN FREE, VEGETARIAN

Very simple
CHOCOLATE MOUSSE

What you need:

3½ ounces/100g dark chocolate (70% cacao), broken into pieces

2 large eggs, separated

2 tablespoons sugar

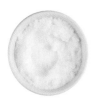

berries and yogurt or whipped cream, to serve

My two favorite words in one name, *simple* and *chocolate*. Craving something sweet when you're low on time can often lead to grabbing an ultra-processed prepackaged treat or digging through whatever desserts are left lurking in the freezer. Prepare this easy, throw-it-together mousse ahead of time and you'll solve the problem beautifully.

How to make it:

• Place the broken-up **dark chocolate** in a heat-safe bowl with ¼ cup/60ml of **water** and set it over a saucepan of simmering water (making sure the bowl does not touch the water). Stir the chocolate from time to time until it's melted, fully combined with the water, and smooth.

• Remove the bowl from the heat and let the chocolate cool for 4–5 minutes. Then stir in the **egg yolks** and set aside.

• Whisk the **egg whites** in a bowl with the **sugar** until stiff. Using a large metal spoon, fold 1 spoonful of the sweetened egg white into the chocolate mixture, and then follow with the rest. Fold gently, so as not to knock out the air from the egg whites.

• Pour the chocolate mousse mixture into four small glasses and refrigerate the mousses for 2–3 hours, until set. Serve topped with some **berries** and a little **yogurt or whipped cream**.

Note: Consuming raw or undercooked meats, poultry, seafood, shellfish, or eggs may increase your risk of food-borne illness.

Makes 4 / Prep time: 25 min, plus setting
GLUTEN-FREE

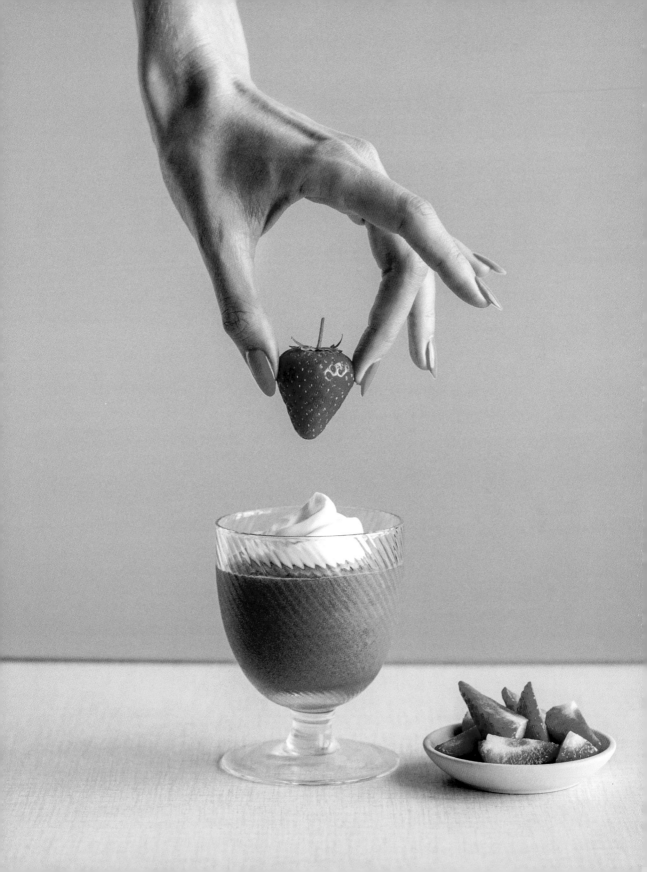

MISO CHOCOLATE TRUFFLES

What you need:

3½ ounces/100g dark chocolate (70% cacao), finely chopped

7 tablespoons/ 100ml heavy cream

1 tablespoon unsalted butter

1 tablespoon white miso (or use brown miso if that's what you have)

1 tablespoon maple syrup

a generous pinch of sea salt

½ cup/60g blanched hazelnuts, roughly chopped

¼ cup/20g cocoa powder

If you've learned anything from this cookbook, besides a plethora of amazing new recipes, of course, I hope it's to expect the unexpected when cooking the Glucose Goddess way. While miso might not be a typical chocolate truffle ingredient, it certainly should be! It's a welcome addition in this dessert that I know you'll adore.

How to make it:

- Place the finely chopped **dark chocolate** in a bowl.

- Pour the **heavy cream** into a small saucepan and add the **butter**. Place the pan on low heat and bring the cream mixture to just below the boiling point.

- When you see the cream start to bubble, remove the pan from the heat and pour the mixture all over the chocolate. Let it rest for a couple of minutes, then stir the mixture until the ganache is smooth and silky.

- Mix the **white miso** and **maple syrup** together, then stir in the generous pinch of **sea salt**.

- Stir the syrup mixture into the chocolate ganache, then stir in the chopped **hazelnuts**. Refrigerate the mixture until it's set (about 2 hours).

- Using your hands, roll the ganache into 15 small truffles, tossing each in the **cocoa powder**. Refrigerate the truffles in a small box, ready for indulging!

Makes: 15 truffles / Prep time: 25 min, plus setting time
GLUTEN-FREE

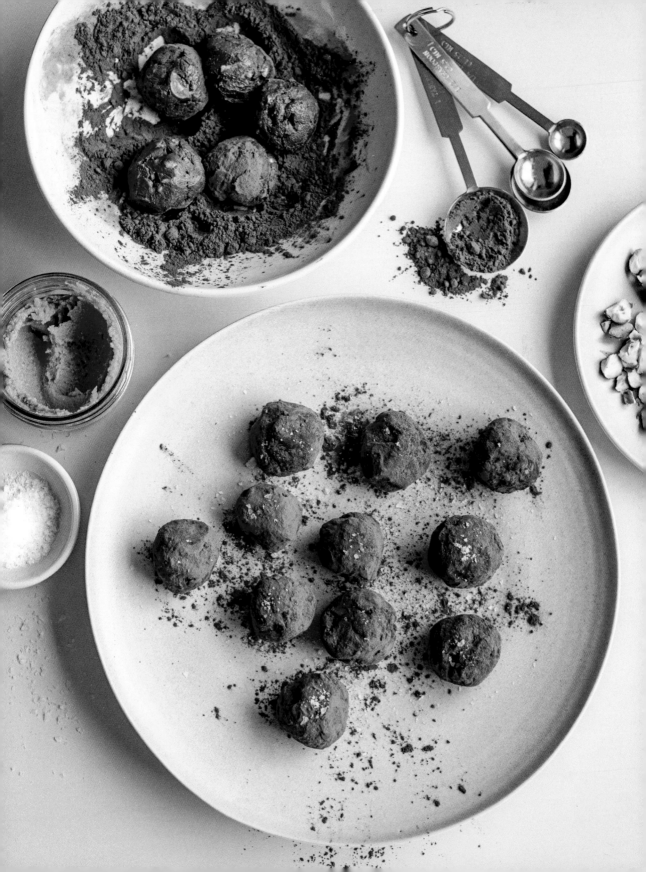

MIXED BERRY *and* PISTACHIO CRUMBLE

What you need:

6 tablespoons /50g all-purpose flour

¾ cup/150g sugar

¼ cup/50g unsalted butter

¾ cup/100g shelled pistachios

2¾ cups/350g frozen mixed berries

crème fraîche, full-fat Greek yogurt, or ice cream, to serve (optional)

Juicy berries with a nutty topping—this crumble is so easy to make. Any frozen berries will work, and you can swap out pistachios for hazelnuts or almonds.

How to make it:

● Preheat the oven to 400°F. Place the **all-purpose flour**, ½ cup/100g of the **sugar**, and the **unsalted butter** in a food processor and blitz until the mixture resembles bread crumbs.

● Add the shelled **pistachios** and blitz again until the nuts are roughly chopped and the crumble has a light green hue.

● Tip the **frozen mixed berries** into a medium round or square baking dish (you want a snug fit) and toss them with the remaining sugar.

● Top the fruit with the nut mixture and bake for 20–25 minutes, or until the berries are bubbling and the crumble is golden and crispy. Serve with crème fraîche, Greek yogurt, or ice cream, if you wish.

Makes: 4 portions / Prep time: 10 min / Total cook time: 25 min
VEGETARIAN

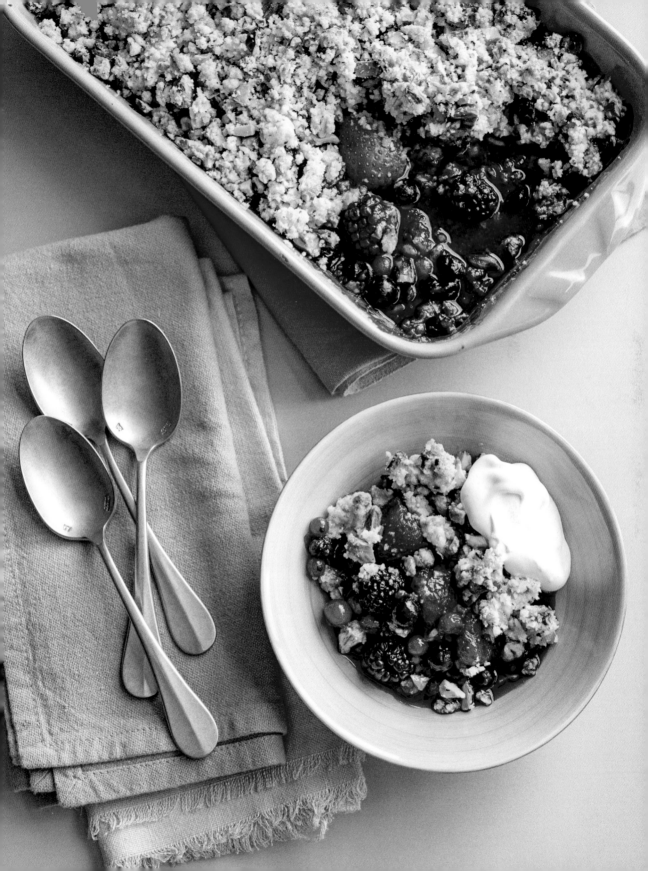

BERRY STEADY ICE CREAM

What you need:

heaping ¼ cup full-fat Greek yogurt

½ cup/100g frozen mixed berries

1 scoop whey protein (or any unflavored and unsweetened protein powder)

1 tablespoon tahini (optional)

An ice cream that will keep your glucose levels steady! You can also enjoy it as an afternoon snack between meals—its balance of low sugar and high protein won't create a spike.

How to make it:

● Spoon the **yogurt** into a plastic tub and place it in the freezer for 3–4 hours, until frozen.

● Transfer the frozen yogurt to a blender along with the **frozen mixed berries**, **whey protein**, and tahini (if using), and blitz. The mixture will become crumb-like to begin with, but keep blitzing and eventually you will have a deliciously smooth, scoopable ice cream. Serve the first portion right away. Freeze the second portion in a freezer-proof container, then either reblend to soften before eating, or simply leave it to soften in the container.

Makes: 2 portions / Prep time: 7 min, plus freezing
GLUTEN FREE, VEGETARIAN

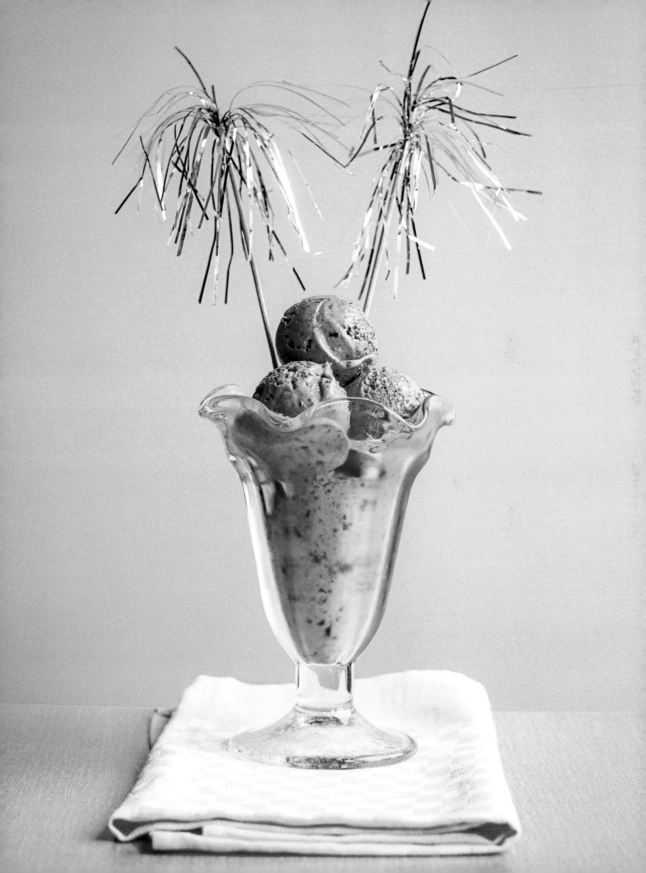

LEMON RICOTTA CHEESECAKE

What you need:

a little butter for greasing the pan

½ cup/100g sugar

1⅓ cups/320g ricotta

3 tablespoons all-purpose flour

3 large eggs, separated

Finely grated zest of 3 unwaxed lemons and juice of 1

1 teaspoon vanilla extract

mixed berries and crème fraîche or full-fat Greek yogurt, to serve (optional)

Lemon ricotta that you'll like a lotta! This cheesecake is so heavenly it'll have you writing poetry about it, too.

How to make it:

● Preheat the oven to 400°F. Line the bottom of a (7-inch/18cm-diameter and 3-inch/7.5cm-deep) springform cake pan with parchment paper. Grease the sides with **butter** and dust the pan with 1 tablespoon of the **sugar**.

● In a bowl, combine the **ricotta**, half of the remaining sugar, the **all-purpose flour, egg yolks, lemon zest** and **juice,** and **vanilla extract** and whisk until smooth.

● In a separate bowl, use electric beaters to whip the **egg whites** until stiff. Add the remaining sugar and beat again until you have a thick and glossy meringue.

● Working very gently, fold the meringue into the ricotta mixture until completely combined.

● Pour the mixture into the prepared pan and bake it on the middle rack of the oven for 35–40 minutes, until golden and risen.

● Remove the pan from the oven and let the cheesecake cool. Then refrigerate it for at least a couple of hours before serving. Serve with some mixed berries and some crème fraîche or Greek yogurt, if you like.

Makes: 6 portions / Prep time: 15 min, plus chilling / Total cook time: 40 min
VEGETARIAN

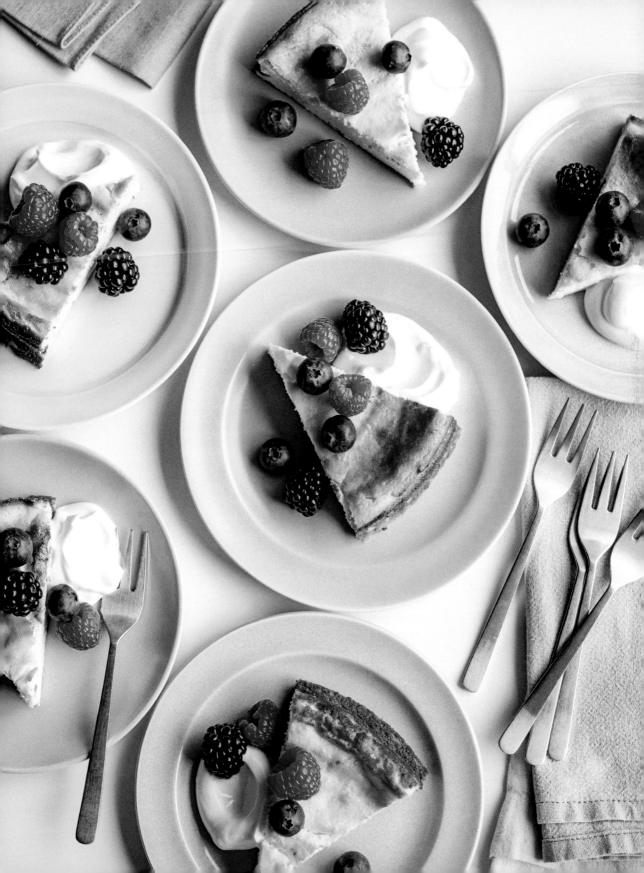

ATOMIC BANANA

What you need:

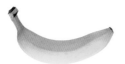

1 ripe unpeeled banana

¼ teaspoon ground cinnamon

1 tablespoon finely chopped walnuts

1 teaspoon tahini (optional)

Watch out! This is going to blow . . . your mind! The Atomic Banana is a well-loved recipe passed down from my Brazilian grandmother. Watching a banana spin and burst in a microwave has remained one of the most exciting things I can think of doing in a kitchen.

How to make it:

● Pierce the peel of the **banana** all over with a fork. Then place the banana on a microwave-safe plate and cook it in the microwave on high for 2 minutes. The banana will burst open and go soft and squishy inside.

● Serve the banana just like that, dusted with **cinnamon**, topped with the chopped **walnuts** and, if using, drizzled with the tahini.

Makes: 1 portion / Prep time: 4 min / Total cook time: 2 min
GLUTEN-FREE, VEGAN

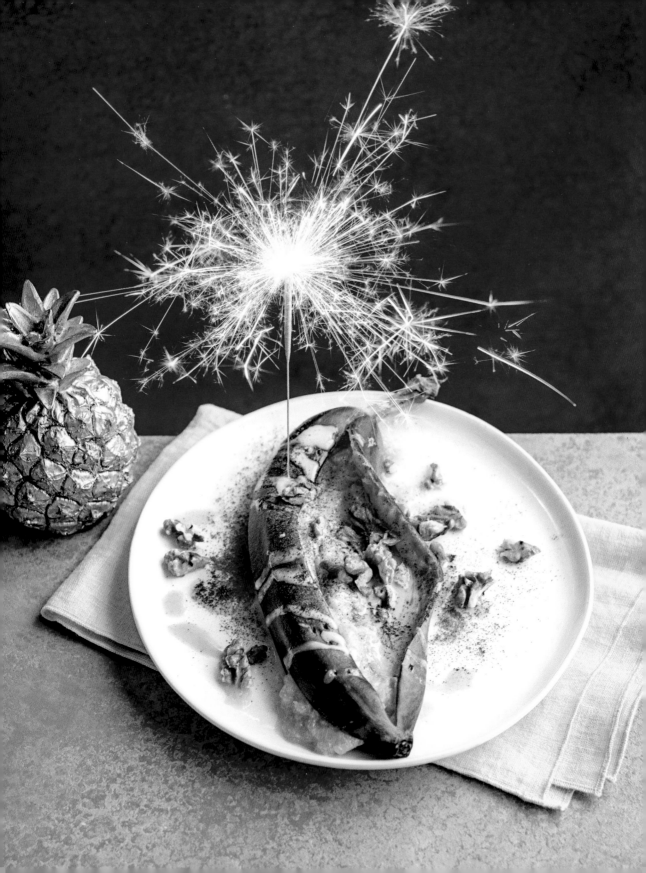

SALTED CHOCOLATE NUT BRITTLE

What you need:

5¼ ounces/150g best-quality dark chocolate (70% cacao), broken into pieces

¼ cup/30g shelled pistachios

3 tablespoons walnut pieces

½ teaspoon sea salt

This dessert is the Glucose Goddess philosophy in a nutshell: very easy and very impressive. And with added fat, fiber, and protein to reduce its spike. Serve it at a dinner party to get admirative "ooohs" and "aahhhs," or keep it to yourself and marvel at its beauty.

How to make it:

● Line a baking sheet with parchment paper. Place the broken-up **dark chocolate** in a heat-safe bowl and set it over a saucepan of simmering water (making sure the bowl doesn't touch the water). Stir from time to time, until the chocolate has melted and is smooth.

● Pour the melted chocolate onto the prepared baking sheet and spread it out to a thin, even layer. Scatter the shelled **pistachios** and the **walnut pieces** all over the melted layer of chocolate and then sprinkle with the **sea salt**.

● Place the baking sheet in the fridge and allow the nutty chocolate to set hard (about 30 minutes).

● Remove the set chocolate from the fridge and break it into bite-size pieces. Keep these ready-to-go treats in an airtight container for up to 2 weeks.

Makes: 1 batch / Prep time: 15 min
GLUTEN-FREE, VEGETARIAN

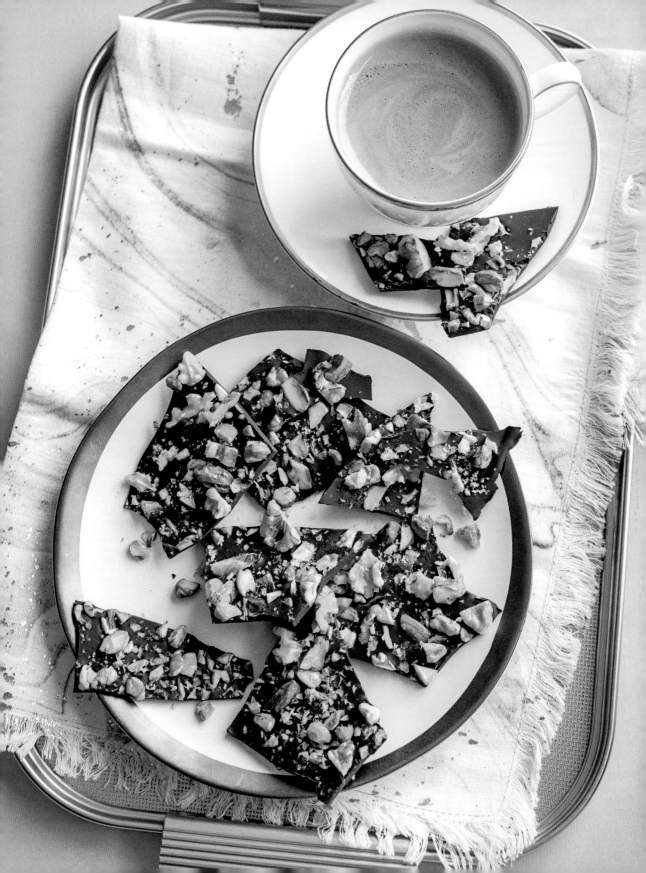

SOS: CRAVINGS

As you flatten your glucose spikes during this Method, your cravings should start to dissipate (because many instances of cravings are as a result of being on a glucose roller coaster). But still having *some* cravings is totally normal. This is a checklist of what to do when you feel one:

First, give your craving a 20-minute cooling-off period. Back in hunter-gatherer days, decreases in our glucose levels signaled that we hadn't eaten in a long time. In response, our brain told us to find tasty foods. Today, when we encounter a decrease in glucose levels, it's usually because the last thing we ate caused a glucose spike. Yet our brain tells us to do the same thing: to choose high-calorie foods, even though we are in no way famished—we've got plenty of energy reserves. After a glucose drop, our liver quickly (within 20 minutes) steps in, releases stored glucose from those reserves into our bloodstream, and brings our levels back to normal. At that point, the craving often dissipates. So next time you're about to grab a cookie, set a timer for 20 minutes. If your craving was due to a glucose drop, it will be gone by the time the alarm rings.

Now check in with yourself: Do you really want to eat this thing, or do you just have the *habit* of eating it? Does your body really want to eat it, or is it an automatic response? This is an important question to ask yourself on your glucose-steadying journey. Stay curious, and allow yourself to update habits if you find that the craving isn't really there anymore.

If it's been 20 minutes and you want to eat the delicious thing, here are some ways of adding a hack to it:

Scenario 1: Eat it now and enjoy it. We don't always want to do hacks, and that's totally normal. I sometimes feel like ice cream for breakfast and that's what I have.

Scenario 2: Eat it, but don't have it on an empty stomach. Set the food you're craving aside and enjoy it as dessert after your next meal. You'll still get the pleasure, but with less impact on your glucose and on your health.

Scenario 3: Put some clothes on it, then eat it. Putting clothes on our carbs and sweets means adding protein, fat, or fiber to an otherwise just starchy and sweet food. For example, have an egg, a handful of nuts, a couple of spoonfuls of full-fat Greek yogurt, or a head of roasted broccoli before the thing you're going to eat.

Scenario 4: Have a vinegar drink before eating the food (see the recipes starting on page 104). The vinegar will reduce the glucose spike of the food and thus you can avoid a cravings roller coaster.

Scenario 5: Use your muscles for 10 minutes after eating the food. Your muscles will soak up some of the glucose as it arrives in your bloodstream and reduce the glucose spike. In the Movement chapter (pages 217–25), I have suggested lots of ideas for how to use your muscles.

You can combine Scenarios 2, 3, 4, and 5 together.

These are some of the glucose-protecting techniques that I keep in the corner of my mind on a daily basis. When it's easy to do so, I add a hack.

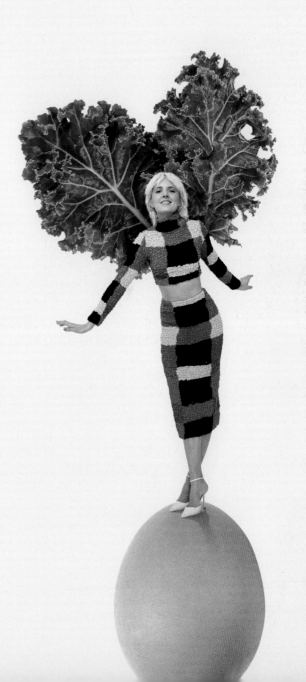

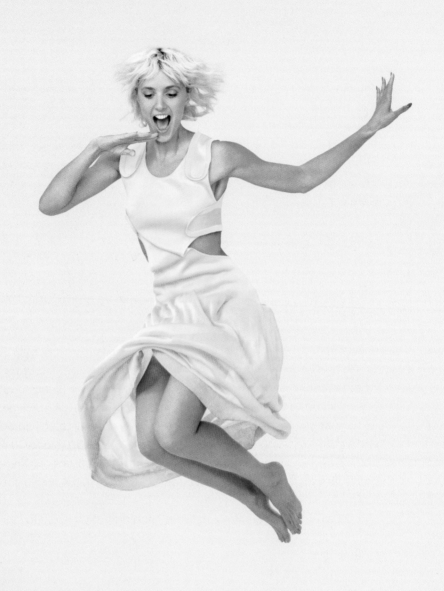

WEEK 4 IS DONE—*now what?*

You did it! Welcome to your future. The year is 3030 and we all have hoverboards.

Just kidding. But the end of this four-week Method *does* kick off the beginning of the rest of your life. Your glucose levels are steadier than ever before; you've unlocked energy, helped your brain, and—I hope—reduced any symptoms you were experiencing.

I also hope that you've connected with your body—that what may have felt like a black box now feels more like a partner that you are getting to know a bit more every day. I hope you have experienced how steadying your glucose levels helps your body and mind thrive and helps you live the life you want to live—and that all you want is to continue to feel better.

Now that you've gotten to know the hacks and they've gotten to know you, they are in your back pocket forever. It's up to you to decide which ones will become daily staples, and which ones will become tools that you can call on when you need them. For most of us, a savory breakfast is now an everyday thing. Vinegar is an ally that we keep in our kitchen and call on before starchy and sweet foods. We've realized that veggie starters are easy to put together, and we always order one when we're out at a restaurant. Moving after eating is a moment that we love coming back to.

I have certainly had an amazing time hanging out with you for these last four weeks. You are now a Glucose God, Goddess, or Nonbinary Deity! I'm pretty sad to leave you, but trust me, we will hang out again soon.

I hope I was a good roommate.

Love, 🖤
Jessie

PS: I watered the plants.

THE PILOT EXPERIMENT PARTICIPANTS

Dear pilot experiment participants, I extend my heartfelt gratitude to you. Because you volunteered to test the Glucose Goddess Method in October 2022 (back when it was still just a PDF), you made it so much better. Your questions informed the program, your ideas improved it, your results are being shared with the world, and your enthusiasm motivated me throughout the process. It was a joy and an honor to connect with you all. As a small token of my appreciation, here are your names (for those of you who wanted your names printed):

Aarthi Balgobind · Abi · Abi Williams · Abigail Baldwin · Abril Escallier · Adela Peralta · Adele Kristensen · Adele Pollard · Aditi Sharma · Adrian Coman · Adriana Dueñas · Adriana Espert · Adriana Pérez P. · Adriana Rebrović · Adrianna Sładek · Adrienn Esik · Adriënne Hazenberg · Aesha Patel · Afton Smith · Aggie · Agnieszka Paszynska · Aidan Belizaire · Aime Broyles · Aimee Waldron · Aimie Guillaume · Ainara Garcia · Alan Zanardi · Alana Calderon · Alba Garrido · Ale Gutierrez Gtz · Alecia Bernardo · Aleena Zahid · Alejandra Corona · Alejandra Torres · Alejandra Vinuesa · Aleksandra Dimitrova · Aleksandra Drewniak · Aleksandra Nazarova · Aleksandra Niemasz · Aleksandra Skierka · Aleksia Aleksieva · Alessandra Peraza · Alessia Del Vigo · Alex Dolly · Alex Lees · Alex Mogck · Alexandra Binder · Alexandra Freemark · Alexandra Lepercq · Alexandra Littwin · Alexandra Pocaterra · Alexandra Tsolakidis · Alexandra Villar · Alexandra Zosimidou · Alexandria Sedar · Alexei Steinmetz · Alexiane Cuenin · Alexis Schüle · Ali Roberts · Ali Smith · Alice Bekima · Alice Kramer · Alice Patin de Saulcourt · Alice Tinaoui · Alice Whitemore · Alicia Esteban · Alicia Zapata · Alina Sliusar · Aline Barré · Aline Borges · Aline Veys · Alisia Humbarger · Alison Elrod · Alison Holcomb · Alison Metcalf · Alissa H. · Alixia Bonte · Allie Ziegler · Allison Bemiss · Alondra Cascante · Alyssa de St. Jeor · Amalia Ileana Pérez Robles · Amalia Módena · Amanda Christenson · Amanda Glidden · Amanda Miller · Amanda Seirup · Amanda Waldon · Amandine Julian · Amandine Poussard · Amanpreet Binner · Amapola Martínez · Ambar Dingemans · Amber Schultz · Amberly Meeker · Amel Alaya · Amelia Diz · Ami-Louise Reid · Amina Syammach · Aminah Husain · Amy Campbell · Amy Carr · Amy Christi · Amy Gingrich · Amy Huff · Amy Johnson · Amy Stewart · Amélie Cosandier · Amélie Martin · Amélie Suire · Ana · Ana Alcañiz · Ana Alejandra Aguayo Topete · Ana B. Rodriguez · Ana Cazacu · Ana Dominguez · Ana Duraes · Ana Ferreira · Ana Fragelli · Ana Garza · Ana Gomes · Ana H. Huembes · Ana I. Longás · Ana Lentino · Ana María Martín González · Ana María Rozo Llanos · Ana Márquez Perrusquía · Ana Paiz · Ana Rodriguez · Ana Vargas · Ana Verónica Portilla Santamaría · Anabell Garcia Cuns · Ananda de Jager · Anastasia Isakova · Anastasia Ivanishchenko · Anastasia Michenko · Anastasija Zubova · Anastazija Dimitrova · Anaëlle Fontaine · Anaïs Arlen · Anaïs D. · Anaïs Radé · Anaïs Rodríguez Villanueva · Andrea Benedicto · Andrea Carrera Flores · Andrea Del Rio · Andrea Hazbun · Andrea Jakes · Andrea Jordà · Andrea Klobučar · Andrea Marroquín · Andrea Miles · Andrea Roussou · Andrea Rubin · Andrea Uribe · Andrea Villegas · Andrea's Brichese · Andreea Cioflica · Andreea Roman · Andressa Colombo · Ane M. Zubizarreta · Ángel Riesgo · Àngela Albert · Angela Bradfield · Angela Edel · Angela Greene · Angela Manasieva · Angela Marasco · Angela Nevin Duffy · Angelica Juarez · Angelica Quintero · Angelika Pryszcz · Angelina Jimenez · Angelo Torrente · Ania Mulica · Ania Verkest · Anil Chawla · Anita Durakovič · Anita Fusiara · Anita Visser · Anja Bajdak · Anja Höft · Anja Wolf · Anjuli Feliciano · Anka Mekota · Ann Boblett · Ann Carr · Ann Moran · Ann-Charlotte Syrén · Anna Anasik · Anna Chipperfield · Anna Dean · Anna Dora · Anna Gloth · Anna Grönfeldt · Anna Haunschmid · Anna Kaczmarczyk · Anna Krysiak · Anna Ludwik · Anna Maisuradze · Anna Nickel-Zelazny · Anna Perez · Anna S. Bendahan · Anna Sarafianou · Anna Sparkz · Anna Wawra · Annabel Stoddart · Annabelle Albany · Annamaria Lookman · Anne Bourboulon · Anne Czerbakoff · Anne Huffman Wall · Anne Tribout · Anne Van Uytven · Anne-Charlotte Quinten · Anne-Laure Soussan · Anne-Lise Fouché · Anne-Sophie Planet · Anneke Greatrex · Annette Cruz · Annette Gardner · Annie Rodriguez · Annie Wood · Annika Jeromin · Anse Mertens · Antoinette Lynch · Antonia Eyzaguirre · Antonia König · Antonia Magdici · Antonio Muñoz · Antsa Raobanitra · Anuar Chehaibar · Aoife McEvoy · Aoife Treacy · Arantxa Mendez Lara · Ariane Preusch · Ashlee Sharrett · Ashleigh Whitmore · Ashley Bailey · Ashley Day · Ashley Graham · Ashley Newman · Ashley Samuelson · Ashley Strahan · Ashlin Shaver · Astrid Grau · Astrid Stevens · Audrey Carette · Audrey Lambert · Audrey Sidot · Auriane Hégron · Aurora Gustafsson · Aurélia Zambaux · Aurélie Govart · Aurélie Mboule · Aviva Halter · Axelle Leclercq · Azouz Amrouche · Balaban Silvia · Barbara Cardoso · Barbara Csutak · Barbara Guffy · Barbara Luarca · Barbara Tierno · Bárbara Yu Belo · Barbora Krupanská · Barbora Viewegh · Bartosz Gackowski · Beatriz Gomez · Beatriz Navarro · Beatriz Pineda · Bec Hill · Becky Bushell · Belén Molaguero · Belén Paniagua · Béatrice Elattar · Béatrice Prevost · Benchy · Benedicte De Jaeger · Beril Geldiay · Bernadeta Pietrzak ·

Bernadett Bohács · Bernadette Zoete · Beth Madeley · Béthianhelle Gioani · Bethsabé Soto · Bettina Lebiu · Bettina Nagy · Bettina Schreck · Bettina Stolz · Bianca Chalfoun · Bianca Meredith · Bianca Nenciu · Bilyana Filiposka · Bilyana Taneva · Bindu Patel · Birgitta Wilson · Birthe Glöß · Blanca Benavides · Bobbie Tootle · Bonni McTighe · Bonnie Troncoso · Bons McLean · Brandi Dorton · Brandi Szoka · Brenda Bailey · Brenda Navarro · Brenda Villapudua · Brittany Lutnick · Brittany Potter · Brittany Walcutt · Brooke Phillips · Bucurenciu Teodora · Caetana Varela-Hall · Caitlin BoWell · Caitlin Imhoff · Caitlin Lakdawala · Caitlin Stooker · Caitlin Vincent · Camarie Naylor · Cameron Wagner · Camila Mondini · Camila Montaldo · Camilla Folci · Camilla Rubino · Camille Flesselles · Camille Toft Knudsen · Camrynne Six · Candela Achával · Capucine de Forton · Capucine Héraud · Cara Meller · Cara Rose Shaw · Caren Yust · Carla Zaffi · Carlotta Della Bella · Carmen Cachafeiro · Carmen Caparrós · Carmen de la Casa · Carmen Haag · Carmen Munteanu · Carmen Schaudt Seyller · Carole Dehlinger · Carole Jagoury · Carole Martelli · Carole Maurel · Carolien Vos · Carolina Alzate · Carolina Bojorquez · Carolina Nazar · Carolina Ochoa · Carolina Pujos · Caroline Bastié · Caroline Demetriou · Caroline Heroufosse · Caroline Hogg · Caroline Janeiro · Caroline Lefebvre · Caroline Marshall · Caroline Mathieu · Carolyn Rodriguez · Carrie Roer · Cassandra Mokdad · Cassandra Smith · Cassie E. Bell · Catalina Rodríguez · Caterina Buonocore · Catharine Anastasia · Catherine King · Catherine Schublin · Cathia Marolany · Cathy Stone · Catia Puhalschi · Cecile Israel · Cecilia Galindo · Cecilia K. · Cecilia Sandoval · Cecylia Go · Chantal Martin · Chantal Uildriks · Charissa Hemmer · Charlene Hanania · Charlie Döring · Charlie Harrison · Charlotte Eberbach · Charlotte Rappleyea · Charlotte Seaton · Charlotte Valdant · Charlène Elizabeth Morel · Chelsea Prugh · Cherie Shepherd · Chiara Del Bene · Chiara Parodi · Chiara Risso · Chiara Rottaro · Chitra Ram · Chloe Stoute · Chloé Caltagirone · Chloé Manca · Chris Seaton · Christa Brasser · Christa Trendle · Christel Simon · Christelle Abougou · Christelle Bordon · Christelle Roblin · Christelle Schaeffer · Christin Hoffman · Christina Cowell · Christina Gellman · Christina Llopis · Christina Perou · Christina Robinson · Christine Gendron · Christine Gray · Christine Guillot-Nion · Christine Lecointre · Christine Rieder · Christy Cluff · Chrysta Musselman · Chyne Chen · Ciara Hoey · Cimpanu Anca Aurelia · Cindy Gendt · Cinthya Abarca Delgado · Cinthya Gonzalez · Cinzia Govender · Citlalli Del Moral · Claire Amo · Claire Churm · Claire Etchells · Claire Humphreys · Claire Khidas · Claire Labbe · Claire Sophie Richwien · Claire Tuytten-Nowak · Clara Estévez · Clara Rousel · Clara S. · Clare Clapp · Clare Howes · Clare Jarvis · Clare Salier · Clare Savage · Clarisa Castrilli · Claudia Belitz · Claudia Canepa · Claudia Haschke · Claudia Romero · Clotilde Hanon · Coline Marchand · Connie DiRenzo · Connie Lipovsek · Constance Boissin · Constanza Elissetche · Coralie Henri-Jaspar · Coralie Vierne · Corina Cepoi · Corina Hébert · Cornelia Hellmer Grahn · Cornelia Popescu · Corrin Campbell · Corrina Horne · Courtenay Cabot · Courtney Blair · Courtney Lawler · Cristina Boix · Cristina Calderaro · Cristina Curto · Cristina Fantin Gatti · Cristina Freitas · Cristina González · Cristina Guizar · Cristina Mingione · Cristina Ordinas · Crystal Gonsalves · Cátia Barros · Cèlia Berenguer · Cécile Breysse · Cécile Brouard · Cécilia Wolfstein · Céline Caillaud · Céline Demmerlé · Céline Ollivier Vincent · Céline Rodrigues · D. Idiart · Damla Hepke · Dana Magyar · Dana Rodriguez · Daniela Albert · Daniela Balderas · Daniela Geneva · Daniela Lugo · Daniela López · Daniela López Estrada · Daniela Martínez · Daniela Maya Sarria · Daniela Sitnisky · Daniela Suárez Elías · Daniela Sánchez García-Reyes · Daniela Wilde · Danielle Bowcut · Danielle Dickson · Danielle Jelfs · Danuzia Carvalho Nunes · Daria Jagielska · Darija Forko · Darya Kryzhanouskaia · Dasha Budkina · Daura Dominguez · Dawn Foxcroft · Dawn James · Dawn Vickers · Dayna Mersberg · Deaf Girly · Deanna Lempi · Debbie Canty · Debbie Cook · Debbie Cox · Debbie Lowe Liang · Debbie Schantz · Deborah Afonso · Deborah Allison · Deborah Freeman · Deborah Griffin · Deborah Nasser · Deborah Van Tuijcom · Debra Rice · Dee Stephenson · Deirdre · Delia Messing · Delphine Houbart · Delzina Assao · Dena Weech · Denise Levine · Denysse Gozalez Ovalle · Desara Rugji · Diana Latvene · Diana McKeag · Diana Pelaez V · Diana Poškienė · Diana Simeonova · Diana Tudor · Diane April · Diane Arnoldy · Diane Gervasi · Diane Jervey · Diane Nguyen · Diane Steffey · Didier Cavasino · Dominique Huyge · Donna Blattel · Donna L. Davidson · Dorina Rozmann · Dorota Rex · Dorothee Flokstra · Dorothy Nordgren · Dulcie Walker · Dóra Veress · Ecklund Leysath · Egle Westerfield · Eileen Loomis · Ekaterina Lyashenko · Elaine Wills · Elena Álvarez · Elena Iglesias · Elena Kummer · Elena Pacchioni · Elena Taelma · Eleni Michael · Eliane Rioux · Elina Rose · Eline Aloy · Elisa Baronio · Elisa Ferreras-Colino · Elisa Laudrin · Elisa M. · Elisa Monti · Elisabeth Smith · Elise Dulova · Élise Herbin · Élise Servan-Schreiber · Elissa Anaya · Elissa Kordulak · Eliza Puna · Eliza Sears · Eliza-Nicoleta Cotocea · Elizabeth Curran · Elke Hein · Ella Sandu · Ellen Capiot · Ellen Dressen · Ellen Garcia Morillo · Ellie · Ellie Richards · Elodie Fosseux · Elodie Palmier · Élodie Saisselain · Eloisa Della Neve · Eloïse Autran · Elsa Pont · Elvira Zebadúa · Elyse Rokos · Ema Dimitrova · Emelie Bonnier · Emeline Thevenon · Emeline Trichet · Emellie Petersson · Emely Taveras Robbs · Emilia Borges · Emilia Kownacka · Émilie Chriqui · Emilie G. · Émilie Nadal · Emilie Thomson · Emily Askea · Emily Hartley · Emily Luong · Emily Minson · Emily O'Hara · Emily Weincek · Emily Williams · Emma Abelsson · Emma Bosher · Emma Colibri · Emma Crocker · Emma Melican · Emmalena Khourey · Erica Woodard · Erika Bustos · Erika Ortega · Erin Jeffers · Erin Sathre · Esperanza Lashi · Esthefanía Latorre G. · Esther Hernández · Esther Poquet · Esther Pugh · Eunice Pérez · Eva · Eva Sissener · Eva Werninger · Eva Zobell · Eve Slegers · Ève Giusto · Éveline Bureau · Evelyn Setubal · Evelyne Van Kerckhove · Evolène Loup · Ewa Adair · Ewa Lenczyk-Chmielarska · Ewa Radziszewska · Fabi Easton · Fabienne Kahne · Fabiola Blake · Fabiola Meza · Famina · Fanchon Roger · Fargier Valérie · Farnaz Beikzadeh · Farrah Khan · Fathima Benazir · Fatima Darago · Fatima Solana · Faustina Maria Giaquinta · Faustine Ankelevitch · Faye Holdert · Fee Naysmith · Felicia Caggiano · Fer Palacios · Fernanda Serna · Fernanda Tomba · Filiz Osman · Filomena Tittarelli · Finnian Coyle · Flavia Eleonora Loretano · Fleur McGregor · Flor Aikawa · Flora Muijzer · Flore Kalfon · Flore Stockman · Florencia Facciuto · Florencia Fernández

Madero · Florencia Girado · Florencia Runco · Franca Mendy · Frances McGeoghegan · Francesca Giambarini · Francesca Marchi · Franciska Stroef · Francka Kozarc · Franziska Moeller · Françoise Leroux · Frederike Hopfenmueller · Frida Uddman · Gabby Hernandez · Gabriela Chacon · Gabriela Figueroa-Sosa · Gabriela Gadsden · Gabriela Hurtado · Gabriela Martinez · Dr. Gabriela Moreno · Gabriela Ramírez · Gabriela Ramirez Rey · Gabriela Sarappa · Gabriela Schuster · Gabriela Welon · Gabriele Gedvile · Gabriella Bachmann · Gabriella Fonseca · Gabrielle · Gabrielle Catti · Gabrielle Lefèvre · Gaby de la Guardia N. · Gaby L. Zapata. · Gaby Meraz · Gael Edwards · Gaelle Henrion · Gaia Aveta De Felice · Gaia Marzi · Gail Solway · Gaylene H. · Gemma Smiddy · Geneva Bondy Noah · Geneviève Cliquet · Genoveva Aretz · Georgia Chrysovergi · Georgiana Boloha · Georgiana Nutu · Georgiana Stanciu · Georgie Pascanu · Georgina Ingram · Geraldine Chell · Gesa Winkens · Ghizlaine · Giada Sera · Gianna Molica-Franco · Gilda Savonitto · Gillian Coleman · Ginger Fox · Giovanna Hummel · Giulia Malachin · Gloria Chea · Grace Henderson · Grace Reinhalter · Grace Rocoffort de Vinnière · Grace White · Graziella Galea · Greta Pearce · Gretchen Bachner · Grethe Lous · Guillermo Gijon Robas · Guilly Willemsen · Gwen Flinsky · Gwenaëlle Page · Hajnal Daniel · Hana Rika Kodela · Hanna Rosinski · Hanna Weckfors · Hanna Woś-Prusak · Hannah Bisig · Hannah Dennerle · Hannah Fasnacht · Hannah Loui · Hannah Orr · Harshita Cherukuri · Hazel Saltis · Heather Atwood · Heather Gray · Heather Greer · Heather Nelson · Hedwig Mabalay-Lawson · Heidi Groom · Helen Byrne · Helen Collins · Helen Gillespie · Helen Pearce · Helen Smith · Helen Wright · Helen Zeus · Helena Casco · Helena Schütte · Helene Virgilan · Helene Vågenes · Henrietta Miller · Hijae Platano · Hilda van Zutphen · Hillary A. Golden · Hélène Bitard · Hélène Lallemand · Hélène Masliah-Gilkarov · Hélène Vasquez · Héloïse Blazy · Holmfridur Sigurdardottir · Iana Kazantseva · Ida Hammerin · Ieva Lukauskaite · Ilana Bergher · Ileana Garcia · Ileana Treviño · Ilona Cuperus · Ilonca Meurs · Imane · Imen Alexandre · Imogen Gater · Imène Abdou · Ina Flavia Sorop · Indre Zakalskyte · Ine Meester · Ines Likeng · Inès Gyger · Inés Comes · Inês Baldaia · Inês de Sousa · Inês Menano · Ingrid Vollmüller · Inma Asensio Crespo · Irazú Corral Pérez · Irem Ersan Ozcifci · Irene Bindels · Irene Chico · Irene de Gruijter · Irene de Roos · Irene McKeagney · Irene Minneboo · Irene Opositares · Irene Palomar · Irina Petrov · Íris Dögg Steinsdóttir · Iris Leon · Iris Piers · Irma Corado · Isa Solal Celigny · Isabel Abel · Isabel De Pauw · Isabel Echeverri Aranzazu · Isabel Máximo · Isabel Rossello Dasca · Isabel Zúñiga · Isabella L. · Isabelle Bouclier · Isabelle Escouboué · Isabelle Fournier · Isabelle Grimm · Isabelle Luberne · Iselin Bay Mjaaland · Iulia Ceparu · Iulia Pascaru · Iva Boneta · Ivana Colo · Ivana Grbić · Ivana Mitrovic · Ivana Zoppas · Ivelina Dekova · Iza Wiśniewska · Izabella Zakrzewska · Jacinta Hennelly · Jackie Gith · Jackie Hernandez · Jackie O'Leary · Jackie Price · Jacque De Borja-Medestomas · Jacqueline L. · Jacqueline Mott · Jacqueline Pulido · Jade Carruthers · Jagruti Kamble · Jaime Regan · Jamie Jensen · Jana Enderle · Jana Peruzzi · Jane Cunningham · Jane Kalme · Janet Slee · Janice Misurda · Janie Shelton · Janin Kortum · Jannemieke Renders · Jannie Postma · Jas Sardana · Jasmin Jabri · Javier Van Cauwlaert · Javiera Bugueño · Javiera Lobos · Jaymee Wise-Tylek · Jayshree Chhatbar · Jazmín Cortes · Jazmin I. Sandoval · Jeanne Adams · Jeanne Lamy-Quique · Jeanne Nolf · Jeanne Wessler · Jelena Volgina · Jen Brown · Jen Eastman · Jen Perkins · Jen Windnagel · Jenette McGiffin · Jenifer Eden · Jenireth Rivero · Jenn Klotz · Jenn Waldron · Jennifer Barwell · Jennifer Brandt · Jennifer Brock · Jennifer González · Jennifer Hunter · Jennifer Menendez · Jennifer Meyer · Jennifer O'Neill · Jennifer Patricia Cariño · Jennifer Smetana · Jennifer Soares · Jennifer Todrani · Jenny Moody · Jess Kennedy · Jessica Bruggeman · Jessica Cherniak · Jessica Coles · Jessica de la Rosa Martínez · Jessica Devine · Jessica Fraser · Jessica Marquardt · Jessica Mast · Jessica Peat · Jessica Taussig · Jessica Tetrault · Jessie Dorrity · Jessie James · Jessie Stupka · Jessika Samryd · Jessy Wearne · Jesús Madrigal Melchor · Jhoana M. Durán · Jill Baxter · Jill Kestner · Jill Marie Anderson · Jill Roberts · Jill Shelley · Jill Summers · Jimena Rodríguez · Jo Breeze · Jo Collyer · Joan Sparks · Joana Caetano · Joana Kriksciunaite · Joana Morais · Joana Samujlo · Joanna Kalisz · Joanne Adams · Joanne Kett · Joanne Pledger · Jocelyne Mingant · Jodi Jones · Jodin Rosales · Jody Scholten · Joe Ciampa · Joesanna Richard · Johanna Engels · Johanna Haarstad · Johanna Schröder · Johanne Royer · John Witten · Jolinda Miller · Joscelin Wreford · Josie Garza · Joséphine L-G · Jovana Bogdanović · Joy Kaminski · Joy Molyneaux · Joy Rainwater · Juan Bland · Jude Curle · Judit González Gayol · Judith Heath · Judith Kay-Cureton · Judith Keys · Judith Rasp · Judith Sorgen · Judy Kealy · Jules Maunder · Julia Astier-Bigot · Julia Dietz · Julia Ganter · Julia Goetsch · Julia Kamel · Julia Knolle · Julia Küpper · Julia Ogrodowczyk vel Ogrodowicz · Julia Oliveira · Julia Wallner · Julia Wilkinson · Juliana Bacelar · Juliana Kontríková · Juliana Milenkovic · Juliana Rossi · Juliana Silva · Julie Alp · Julie Clabeau · Julie Crisinel · Julie Delé · Julie Dobish · Julie Draper · Julie Dreno · Julie Gaudin · Julie Hargraves · Julie Marie Ramirez · Julieta García · Julieta Paganini · Juliette Canard · Juliette Cousin · Julio Benitez · Juncal Ruiz · Justyna Mroczek · Justyna Szachowska · K. Adams · Kaan Kaya · Kaisa Grosjean · Kallisto Papaioannou · Kamila Chilewski · Kamila Lípová · Kamilla Cospen · Karen Adler · Karen Banducci · Karen Berger · Karen Churchill · Karen DeGrazio · Karen Goodliffe · Karen Hill · Karen Self · Karen Smith · Karen Tapia · Karen Watson · Karin Junger · Karin Lummis · Karin MacKinnon · Karina Galiano-Nussbaumer · Karine Marianne · Karis Howard · Karla Arevalo · Karla Fierro · Karla Venegas · Karolina · Karolina Spustova · Karolina Łagosz · Karolina Łuczkiewicz · Karyn Hughes · Kasia Bond · Kasia Mitura · Kat Kimber · Kat McS · Katarina Đozović · Katarina Jovanovic · Katarina Markic · Katarina Sahlin · Katarzyna Konieczna · Kate Bowdren · Kate Bowsher · Kate Rivett · Kate Stanford · Kate Stockwell · Kath Lewis · Katharina Molzahn · Katharina Schaber · Katharina Stanasiuk · Katharine Daly · Katherina Reich · Kathleen Seco · Kathrin · Kathrin Schirazi-Rad · Kathrin Schmid · Kathryn Beesley · Kathryn Gouveia · Kathryn Rees · Kathryn Watson · Kathy Calvo · Kathy Farrell · Kathy Palacios · Kati Vellak · Katia Caillou · Katia Nicolas · Katie Anderson · Katie Benjamin · Katie Booth · Katie

Fenstemaker · Katie James · Katie Kouchi · Katy Jourdannet · Katy Segal · Katy Syme · Katya Chertkova · Kayla Oeyma · Kaylan Miller · Kayleen Steel · Kelly Brinkman · Kelly Bruxvoort · Kelly Gordon · Kelly Koplin · Kelly Ten · Kelsey Low · Kera Hayden · Keri Yother · Kerry · Kerry Hardy · Kerry Wilson · Kerstin Healy · Kerstin Lesen · Keylor Sánchez · Keziah Austin · Khadija Marchoud · Kim Barnett · Kim Budden · Kim Myers · Kim Sotir · Kimara Solomon · Kimber Westmore · Kimberlee Daugherty · Kimberly Henry Cobb · Kimberly Rofrano · Kinga Łobejko-Janik · Kinsey Mead · Kira Lewis · Kirsten Rincon · Kirsten Vermaak · Klaudia Kijas · Klaudia Zyla · Klementyna Dec · Klementyna Ziomek · Kris Ledesma · Kris Naglich · Krissy Whittenburg · Kristen Hunt · Kristen Smyth · Kristen York · Kristi Downs · Kristi Solt · Kristín Bjarnadóttir · Kristin Matuszewski · Kristin Rowland · Kristin Vergouwen · Kristina Busilaitė · Kristina Danchevska · Kristina Luković · Kristina Rastauskienė · Kristine Walton · Kristyna Zlesakova · Kseniia Rozhko · Kyla Marshall · Kylee Bryan · La Goulip · LaDonna Steele · Laetitia Monvoisin · Laetitia Routin · Lahari Kolanupaka · Lara Bello · Lara Mambuay · Lauma Rafelde · Laura Arenas · Laura Benouari · Laura Bineviciute · Laura Bishop · Laura Camilleri · Laura Campos Velasquez · Laura Carretero · Laura Cavaliere · Laura Chávez · Laura Comte · Laura Echavarría · Laura Eik · Laura Foster · Laura Gallon · Laura Gil · Laura Hecht · Laura Hotchkiss · Laura Janssen · Laura Klimmek · Laura Kramer · Laura Machuca · Laura Seibt · Laura Smet · Laura Vanbellinger · Laura Waite · Laura Weiland · Laure Journeau · Laurel Moore · Lauren Baker · Lauren Floore-Guetschow · Lauren Kato · Lauren Polson · Lauren Rappleyea · Lauréna Emmanuel · Laurence Biboud · Laurence Cauvy · Laurence Girouard · Laurence Mourot · Laurent Amar · Lauriane Boucher · Laurie Scheinman · Laverne Swanepoel · Lazarina Peneva · Léa Choichit · Léa Salgado · Leah Eberhardt · Leah Nielson · Leanne Charlton · Leanne Paluch · Leanne Strachan · Leda Rivero · Lee Wiebe · Lee-Sara Davis · Legia Oswald · Lena Grab · Lena Hofbauer · Lena Smets · Lesley Charnick · Lesley Pringle · Lesli Grace Medina · Leslie Fernandez · Leslie Ramirez · Leslie Skolnik · Leyla Prézelin · Līga Rozīte · Lila Jonsson · Lila Jurado · Lilia Chairez · Lilja Lior Polak · Lina Aarnio · Linda Lonsdale · Linda Reece · Linda van Mierlo · Linda Zucker · Lindsay Hindman · Lindsey Comber · Lindsey Ecker · Lindsey Smith · Lindy Graham · Lisa Betzler · Lisa Bice · Lisa Chamberland · Lisa Dhoop · Lisa Harris · Lisa Lipari · Lisa Milner · Lisa Nowak · Lisa Ryan · Lisa Shub · Lisa Tucker · Lisa Vieweg · Lisa Weidinger · Lisa Widener · Lisete Andre Cleary · Lison Génot · Lisseth Naranjo · Liz O'Nions · Liz Rainbow · Liz Smith · Liza Juliana Suárez Rincón · Lois Allen · Lois Howard · Loly Arellano · Lorelee Ljuboja · Lorelei Kelly · Lorena Neira · Lorens Ripoll · Lorenza Mazzone · Lori Stevens · Lou Deyn · Lou-Ann Mir · Loubna Chaoui · Louisa Scott · Louise Hetherington · Louise Hutchings · Louise Johnson · Louise Quinn · Louise Searson · Louise Sklar · Louise Smith · Louise Valentine · Louise van den Broek · Louise Wallet · Louise Wetenkamp · Lourdes Norzagaray · Anabela Nunes-Edwards · Loz Cha · Luba Martemyanova · Lucelly Gonzalez · Lucia Guajardo · Lucía Sández · Lucia Solorzano · Lucía Vazquez · Luciana Battistessa · Lucie Morel Collette · Lucie Rebillard · Lucila Macadam · Lucile Dahan · Lucile Robert · Lucille Valentin · Lucinda Ciciora · Lucy Ruffier · Ludivine Cherif-Cheikh · Ludovica Zorzetto · Luis Araujo · Luísa Buogo · Luisa Estrada-Mallarino · Luisa Nodari · Luli Cadenas · Luz María Aragón · Lydia Djender · Lydia Gerritsen · Lydia Vian · Lydie Morin · Lyndall Metherell · Lynn Pulford · Lynne Elliott-Dawson · Lynne Harrop · M. Daniela Salas · Maaike Teunis-Mudde · Macarena Urzúa · Macarena Vergara · Madalynn Spiller · Madeline A B P · Madison Lovo · Madison Satterfield Mathis · Mafe Agudelo · Magali Duquenoy · Magali Minond · Magalie Nkiani · Magda Bednarczyk · Magda D'Andrea · Magdalena Pappalardo · Magdalena Radosaveljevic · Mai Wong · Maija Milbrete · Maite Hontiveros-Dittke · Maja Alivojvodić · Majda · Majida Husseini · Malgorzata Block · Malgorzata Nowicka · Manahil Saber · Mandie Smith · Mandy de Bruijn · Mandy Peeling · Mandy Whitaker · Mar Cano · Mara Nelson · Marcela Cazenave · Marcela Cotes-Connolly · Marcela Mitrano · Marcela Roberson · Marci Boland · Marcia Darinthe · Mareike Schmidt · Margarita Ludlow · Margaux Liebmann · Mari Carmen Parra · Maria A. Piedrahita · Maria Adelaida Quitero Mesa · Maria Alejandra Giraldo · Maria Butler · Maria Campuzano · Maria Carolina Osorio · Maria Casas · Maria Clara Ribeiro de Lima · Maria Claudia Moreno · Maria Fernanda Peña Prieto · Maria Isabel Caicedo · Maria Lippold · Maria Malcisi · Maria Marta Castillo · Maria Melis · Maria Mendez · Maria Mercedes Agudelo · Maria Newkirk · Maria P. · Maria Paula Olaya · Maria Pietrzak · Maria Tangarife · Maria Vittoria Rosa · Mariah Vigil · Mariah Virden · Mariam Abrahamyan · Mariana Corzo · Mariana Fernandes · Mariana Ramírez-Degollado · Marianthi Tsitlaidi · Maribel Villa · Maricarmen Aguilar · Marie · Marie Paiser · Marie Pinart · Marie Vanbremeersch · Marie Wagner · Marie-Aude Blakeway · Marie-Eugénie Laurent · Marie-Pierre Deshayes · Marie-Pierre Dura-Swiderski · Marie-Sara Vigouroux · Marija Kontrimaite · Marija Zorić · Marilena Sapienza · Marilyn Morales Mora · Marina Dorn · Marina Todorovic · Marina Zărnescu · Marine Aznar · Marine Maize · Marine Quilichini · Marion Baniant · Marion Depéry · Marion Jentsch · Marion Mauvoisin · Marion Richter · Marion Schmidt · Mariquiña Gómez · Marisa Arroyo · Marisa Asheim · Marissa Schwent · Marit Nordstad · Marit Oosterwijk · Marjelle Alkema · Marjolaine Taussat · Marjorie Sburlino · Marla Glabman · Marlene Molina · Marlina Sol · Marloes Albers · Marloes Wolkenfelt · Marlous Bertens · Marni Levy · Marta Candeias · Marta Causapé · Marta Chiesa · Marta González · Marta Guarch · Marta Haering · Marta Rajca · Marta Rędowicz · Marta Yustos · Marta Zielinska · Martha Cortez · Martha Félix · Martin Huschka · Martina Đođo · Martine de Graaf · Marty Barbui · Maru Schulz · Maru Villarreal · Mary Ann Welch · Mary Ciampa · Mary Coates · Mary LaBuz · Mary Mayne Moore · Maryam Krupa · Mary-Anne Osborne · Maryann Pellegrini · María Bausili · María Deleito-Campos · María Elena Nieto Pena · María Fernanda Liñares · María Luengo García · María Paula Bustos Moreno · María Pazos · MaríaJosé Jorquera · Mas-udah Essop · Mathilde · Mathilde Thin · Mattea Romani · Maura Cullum · Maura Martinez · Maureen White · Mayra Fernandes · Mayra Quevedo Cardoso · Maïa Birn · Maïté Bellet-

Wedgwood · Maÿlis Puyfaucher · MC Casal · Meagan Rogers · Meagan Toulouse · Mechi Ginzo · Meg Hoke · Megan Barrett · Megan Goodwin · Megan Julio · Megan Moniz · Mei Ling Giada Jang · Melanie Bichler · Melanie Mauldin · Melanie Terrill · Melina Glogger · Melinda Antol · Melissa Boddaer · Melissa Bommarito · Melissa Bradford · Melissa Daenzer · Melissa LaRoche · Melissa Lot · Melissa Morrison · Melissa Rodarte · Melissa Scott · Melissa Shepherd · Melissa Vassenelli · Mendy van de Ven · Meral Diepeveen · Merari Medellín · Mercedes Rivero · Mercedes Velarde · Meredeth Flores · Meredith Tracy · Merel Holtrop · Merriam Conte · Micaela Bartolucci Cuacci · Michaela Kastelovicova · Michaela Koch · Michaela Landau · Michaela Maier · Michela Pola · Michele Kelly · Michele Michaeli · Michele Sullivan · Michele Weatherford · Dr. Michelle A. Caban-Ruiz · Michelle Aregger · Michelle C. · Michelle Ciavola · Michelle Cleary · Michelle van Beek · Michelle Vargas · Michelle Wingfield · Micu Andreea · Miguel Figueroa · Mihaela Indricean · Mila Martín · Milagros Meléndez · Milena Sokolic · Milla Suvikannel · Mille Toft Sørensen · Mina Kalina · Mirana Lince · Miriam Fernandez-Mendez · Miriam Outabarrhist · Mirona Grzybowska · Missy Beach · Mitra Buicki · MJ Feeke · Moira Sananes · Mollie Mubeen · Monica Cao · Monica Ghenta · Monica Prieto · Monica White · Moniek de Ruijter · Monika Dabrowska · Monika Kurek · Montse Juárez · Morgane Duval · Mouna Rabih · Munera Adel · Muriel Bad · Muriel Eberlin · Muriel Mureau · Mylène Colombat · Myriam Chebbi · Méghane Favrel · Mélanie Caspar · Mélanie D. Vendette · Mélanie Lemmens · Mélanie Vallas · Nadezhda Todorova · Nadia Cantisani · Nadia Janssens · Nadia Roessler · Nadina Duma · Nadiya Bazlyankova · Naiara Martín · Nancy Ocampo · Nancy Rudolph · Nani Glover · Nanna Browning · Naomi Kambere · Naomi Vingron · Nashira Yanez · Natacha Licata · Natacha Marin Lindez · Natalia Gutiérrez Támara · Natalia Janowicz · Natalia Maczka · Natalia Novoa · Natalia Rostova · Natalie Baxter · Natalie Berthiaume · Natalie Franz · Natalie Frisby · Natalie Gaulin · Natalie Kaar · Natalie Palmer · Natasha Cabral de Lacerda · Natasha Kuchinski · Nataša Mandić · Nathalie Alvarez · Nathalie Badin · Nathalie Bourgeois · Nathalie Erbrech · Nathalie Feliu · Nathalie Michaux · Nathalie Peyre · Navneeta Pathak · Nellie Hill · Neoshi Chhadva · Nerina Keiner · Nesrina Schweizer · Nevena Banovic · Neža Tepina · Nichole Crawford · Nichole Peasley · Nichole Sorenson · Nicola Kelly · Nicole Behrens · Nicole Burpo · Nicole Cantrell · Nicole Couto · Nicole Kas · Nicole Offerman · Nicole Saad · Nicole Weigel · Nicole Wielandt · Nicolette Ardelean · Nika Štrus · Niki VanValkenburg · Nikki Pearson · Nikolina Mihaylova · Nils H. Johansson · Nina Bate · Nina Craig · Nina Gaggiano · Nina Pahor · Nina Thörnqvist · Nisaa Seedat-Motlekar · Niyati Seth · Noe Ortega · Noemi Burgos · Nora Benneter · Nora Centioni · Nora Noske · Nora Sandig · Nora Tomac · Noreen Dowling · Norma Ghamrawi · Nour Boukhari · Oana-Raluca Miclea · Odessa Tseng · Ola Jacukowicz · Olga Aguilar · Olga Bellido · Olga Bergmann · Olga Fidalgo · Olimpia Yepez · Olivia Battisti · Olivia Maida · Olivia Salvia · Olivia White · Olívia Hancová · Oriana Ceffa · Oriana Rossi · Ornella Bernardi · Osvelia Ramírez · Page Peoples · Paloma Hidalgo · Paloma Lopez · Paloma Sánchez · Pamela Assandri · Pamela Brotherton · Pamela McGeachan · Pamela Rivera · Pamela Valerio · Paola Colesnik · Paola Della Rocca · Paola Esteves · Paola Rodríguez Guaba · Paola Stellari · Pascale Weber · Pat Volza · Patricia Consales · Patricia Estrada · Patricia Knebel · Patrícia Rodrigues · Patricia Rodríguez · Patricija Pabalytė · Patrick Hudson · Patrizia Fusco · Patti Jo Capelli · Patti Wilcox · Paula Álvarez · Paula Bock · Paula Capodistrias · Paula García · Paula Méndez González · Paula Reisen · Paula Sanin · Paulina Amador · Paulina Carlström · Paulina Galka · Paulina Mendez · Pauline Chabert · Pauline Lula Dagron · Pauline Mahu · Pauline Ott · Pavlina Reka · Peggy Calmettes · Peggy Kierstan · Penny Eubanks · Petra Chappell · Petra Zborilova · Petya Stankova · Philippine Marle · Phillipa Selfe · Pholisa Fatyela · Pia-Celina Stang · Pim Sottomayor · Pola Capuano · Polona Juricinec · Prisca Salaï · Priscilla Cruz · Priscilla Moradel · Priscillia Treacy · Priya Patel Sathe · Priyanka Sadhu · Quinn Walsh · Rachael Chandler · Rachael Dean · Rachel Blair · Rachel Cook · Rachel Cornet · Rachel Ilett · Rachel Kruse · Rachel Macleod · Rachel Park · Rachel Sherve · Rachel Simmet · Rachel Thokala · Rachel Utain-Evans · Rada Kemilova · Radhia Alvi · Rafaela I. · Rafaela Sinopoli · Raffy · Raïssa Ronda · Raluca Lupulescu · Raluca Najjar · Randa El Dirini · Randi Sternberg · Rani Russy · Ratna Mamidala · Raziye Akilli · Rebeca Coman · Rebecca Bloor · Rebecca Finsterwalder · Rebecca H. · Rebecca L. · Rebecca Lowrance · Rebecca Olave · Rebecca Ottusch · Rebecca Pulliam · Rebeka Pregelj · Regina Gruden · Regina Loft · Regina Nielsen · Regina Solomon · Renata Dibou · Renate Prees · Resham Shah · Rey Campbell · Rhea Ghotgalkar · Rhianne Pearson · Rhym Abdennbi · Rica Schlegel · Rietha Mueller · Riëtte Cawthorn · Rima Linaburgyte · Roberta Green · Robin Caceres · Robin Matheny · Robyn Butler · Robyn Heynes · Rocio Martin · Rocio Villagra · Rocío Corso · Rocío Saborido · Rod Hutchings · Roisin Kanupp · Roma Lakhani · Romane Pierrot · Romina Rueda · Ron Domingo · Ronda Ruckman · Rosa Crespo · Rosa Crespo Sanchidrian · Rosa May · Rosalie El Awdan · Rosana Festa · Rose Evans · RoseMarie Jensen · Roser Pellicer · Rossella De Angelis · Roxana Knies · Roxana Treviño-Wilson · RoxAnne Tierney · Roz B. · Rozanne Stevens · Rubaiya Hussain · Rusudan Martirosyan · Ruth González · Ryanne den Ouden · S. Andert · Sabina van Boxtel · Sabina van der Heijden · Sabine Mosca · Sabrina Kress · Sabrina Mahrougui · Sabrina Silva · Sabrina Stiller · Sabrina Wouters · Sabrine Stabile · Sadia Awan · Safa Awad · Sally Bricker · Sally Buchanan Nicol · Sally Cordier · Sally Higgs · Sally Turney · Salma Belouah · Salomé Diament · Sam Wright · Samah Zarif · Samantha Burroughs · Samantha Epstein · Samantha Griffiths · Samantha Gutierrez · Samantha Hipperson · Samantha Moss · Sandi Minneci · Sandra Aguilar · Sandra Chabrerie · Sandra Chavez · Sandra Durakovic · Sandra Klipn · Sandra Petri · Sandra Vallecillo · Sandra Yates-Smith · Sandrine de Meyer · Sandrine Debetaz · Sandrine Deliaud · Sandrine Duclos · Sandy Gill · Sanju Shampur · Sanna Ljungqvist · Sanne Hopman · Santiago Bedoya · Sara Archer · Sara Cameron · Sara Cangelosi · Sara Canullo · Sara Dias · Sara Freitas · Sara Gardner · Sara Kelley · Sara Krdzavac · Sara L. Oliver · Sara Lenzi ·

Sara McGrath · Sara Miguel · Sara Polanc · Sara Shoemake · Sara Willmore · Sarah Bouziane · Sarah Brunton · Sarah C. · Sarah Cohen Valle · Sarah Cooper-Gadd · Sarah Delang · Sarah Ellis · Sarah Evison · Sarah Ford · Sarah Gee · Sarah Habri · Sarah Hartmann · Sarah Johnson · Sarah K. Weiss · Sarah K.-T. · Sarah Kahn · Sarah Nunes · Sarah Pandoursky · Sarah Rayner-Royall · Sarah Rossiter · Sarah Seely · Sarah Slizovitch · Sarah Turner · Sarah Wagner · Sarah Waite · Sarah-Rose Muldoon · Saralina Barragan · Sarolta György · Sasha Rashid · Saskia Burauen · Saskia van Ewijk · Savanna Brady · Savanna Marsicek · Savannah Ball · Selin Okunak · Sergia Maria Schiratti · Shanda Metzinger · Shanna Vasquez · Shannon DeLello · Shannon Grzybowski · Shannon Spaulding · Sharisa Lewis · Sharon Bosch · Sharon Humphrey · Shasta Garcia · Shauna Perger · Sheila Dominguez · Shelby Falk · Shelley Herron · Shelley Martel · Shelley Sonand · Shelli Kennedy · Shermila Paula · Sherri Robertson · Shilpa K K · Shonda Palmer · Shonette Bason · Shonna Menzo · Shpresa Sadiku · Sibilla Rižova · Sidonie André · Sigrid Jochems · Silja Neisskenwirth · Silvana Gonzalez Capria · Silvia Castelan · Silvia Solé · Simina-Larisa Iancu · Simona Balaban · Simona Braileanu · Simone Broos · Simran Mann · Sina Perez · Sinéad Burke · Siobhan Burke · Siobhán Hallissey · Sirma Tsvetkova · Sissel Gram Warringa · Sittana Abdelmagid · Siyavuya Vukutu · Slava De Gouveia · Sneha Somaya · Snæfríður Pétursdóttir · Sofia BAM · Sofia Camargo · Sofía Giubergia · Sofia Murarus · Sofía Pardo · Sofía Ramos · Sol Magana · Sonia García · Sonia Jerez · Sonia Kaminska · Sonia Santana · Sonja Lewis · Sonya Stocker · Sophie Andrews · Sophie Cherry · Sophie Gétaz · Sophie Kenneally · Sophie Koet · Sophie L. · Sophie Mouton · Sophie Reinwarth · Sophie Saulnier · Sophie Schirmer · Sophie Schyns · Sorana V. · Soraya Moussaoui · Soreya Dessai · Špela Čuk · Špela Koštrun · Stacey Freier · Stacey Noah · Stacia Hanley · Stacie Mackay · Stefani Peters · Stefanie Dellepiane · Stefanie Grayeski · Stéfanie Mercier · Stefanie Panhuyzen · Stefanie West · Steffi · Stela Dimitrova · Stella Kirby · Steph Moran · Stephania Solano · Stephanie Cutlip · Stephanie Dion · Stephanie Gao · Stephanie Guinn · Stephanie Kaiser · Stephanie Lois · Stephanie Martire · Stephanie St. Hill · Stephanie Whalen · Stojanka Palko · Stuthi Vijayaraghavan · Stéphanie Belrose · Stéphanie Reimat · Stéphanie Salvador · Sue Hara · Sunmy Jo · Susan Arbing · Susan Hammer · Susan Kilmer · Susana Conde · Susana Salazar · Susannah Bleakley · Susie KB · Susie Morrison · Suzanne Bahls · Suzanne Giblett · Suzanne Jekel · Suzanne O'Dowd · Suzanne Owens · Suzica · Suzie Coucher · Suzie Murphy · Suzy Tenenbaum · Svetlana Krassa · Sydney Cruz · Sylina Sabir · Sylvia Stoyanova · Sylwia Oakley · Székely Tímea · Tabatha Villarroel · Talia Laird Wasch · Talia Siller · Tamara Diaz-Varela · Tammy de Nobrega · Tammy Russell · Tammy Warner · Tamrin de Robillard · Tania Briceño · Tania Searle · Tania Yunes · Tanja Sørfjord · Tanya Henley · Tanya Merriott · Tanya Sutton · Tatiana Infante · Tatiana Ketelbuters · Taylor DaSilva · Taylor Naber · Taylor Roakes · Telva Mejia · Teodora Tănase · Teresa Lima · Teresa Pimentel · Teresa Villanueva Delgado · Teresita Carrasco · Teri Willis · Terri Kluck · Terry Holmes · Tess Tegenbos · Thalyssa Duarte · Thaís Linguanotto · Theresa Vaccari · Thirza Parton · Tiffany Singh · Tiia Neeme · Tijana Pljakic · Tijana Veljković · Tina Rice · Tina Scheliga · Tina Sedigh Mirazimi · Tina Turnbull · Tiziana T. · Tonia Collett · Tonia Devolder · Toota Maher · Tova Nathanson · Tracy Bermeo · Tracy Matthews · Tregaye Lacey · Tricia Honey · Tricia Wilkins · Trisha Helms · Triza Mihigo · Tsvetina Vekova · Tsvetomila Toncheva · Tullia Santorin · Tynley Bean · Tícia Knap · Ula Miśko · Ulrike Brucher · Unam Arshad · Ursula Gradl · Ursula Guilfoyle · Urvi Thakkar · Vaiva Miliukaite · Valentina Indino · Valentina Riva · Valeria Bodò · Valeria Myklebust · Valeria Pace · Valeria Rijana · Valerica Mihai · Valerie Artrip · Valérie Cormier · Valerie Steisslinger · Valeriia Prydvor · Vanessa Cruz · Vanessa Farfán · Vanessa Milewski · Vanessa Sears · Vanessa Vetencourt · Vanina Franco · Verity Jones · Vero López Barrios Acuña · Vero Seguí · Veronica Anica · Veronica Martin · Veronica McBride · Verónica Miguel · Verónica Monge Gómez · Veronica Wintoneak · Veronika Vidic · Véronique Palma · Veronique Tutenel · Vesela Kostova · Vicki Goodsell · Vicki Kehres · Vicky Balliere · Vicky Ribbens · Victoria · Victoria Herrera · Victoria Holtby · Victoria Milbrath · Victoria Monod · Victoria O'Brien · Victoria Yao · Viktoria Szeles · Vilma Zigmantaitė · Vini B. · Vinice Cowell · Vino Lakshminarasimhan · Viola Lutchman · Violeta Petkov · Virginia Evans · Virginia Mena R. · Virginia Riva · Virginie Boittiaux · Virginie Palliser · Virginie Souverain · Vita Trkulja · Viviana Lobos · Vivien Hamed · Vivienne May · Višnja Tasić · Wafa Sahil · Wafaa Amin · Wajeeha MKhan · Wendy Lane · Wendy R. Raymond · Weronika Łapka · Whitney Morrison · Whitney Swander · Wies van Lieshout · Wiktoria Czyż · Xanthia Walker · Xchel Palafox · Xennia Montoya · Xhenete Ramadani · Xiomara Del Rio · Yagna Beltran · Yara Yung · Yasmin Andraca · Yaël Grossmann · Yelena Garcia · Yiviani Estrada · Yolanda Aguilera · Yolanda Perez · Yurany Del Castillo · Yvonne Woods · Zannatul Akter · Zelipah Mitti · Zerimar Gonzalez · Zofia Wójcik · Zohra Jebari · Zoi Montatore · Zoë Van Daele · Zuzanna Czolnowska · Zuzanna Michalewicz

SCIENTIFIC REFERENCES

In my first book, *Glucose Revolution*, I noted the 300+ scientific papers that support my work. These papers also serve as the basis for this book. On this page, I have noted further sources that I have referenced to write *The Glucose Goddess Method*. If you'd like to see all the scientific references, head to: www.glucosegoddess.com/science.

Poor sleep

St-Onge, Marie-Pierre, Anja Mikic, and Cara E. Pietrolungo. "Effects of diet on sleep quality." *Advances in Nutrition* 7.5 (2016): 938–949, https://pubmed.ncbi.nlm.nih.gov/27633109/.

Tsereteli, Neli, et al. "Impact of insufficient sleep on dysregulated blood glucose control under standardised meal conditions." *Diabetologia* 65.2 (2022): 356–365, https://link.springer.com/article/10.1007/s00125-021-05608-y.

Mood

Bushman, Brad J., et al. "Low glucose relates to greater aggression in married couples." *Proceedings of the National Academy of Sciences* 111.17 (2014): 6254–6257, https://www.ncbi.nlm.nih.gov/pmc/articles/PMC4035998/.

Strang, Sabrina, et al. "Impact of nutrition on social decision making." *Proceedings of the National Academy of Sciences* 114.25 (2017): 6510–6514, https://www.pnas.org/doi/10.1073/pnas.1620245114.

Swami, Viren, et al. "Hangry in the field: An experience sampling study on the impact of hunger on anger, irritability, and affect." *PLoS One* 17.7 (2022): e0269629, https://pubmed.ncbi.nlm.nih.gov/35793289/.

Brain fog

Takahashi, Hironori, et al. "Glycemic variability determined with a continuous glucose monitoring system can predict prognosis after acute coronary syndrome." *Cardiovascular Diabetology* 17.1 (2018): 1–10, https://pubmed.ncbi.nlm.nih.gov/30121076/.

Watt, Charles, Elizabeth Sanchez-Rangel, and Janice Jin Hwang. "Glycemic variability and CNS inflammation: Reviewing the connection." *Nutrients* 12.12 (2020): 3906, https://pubmed.ncbi.nlm.nih.gov/33371247/.

Yang, Junpeng, et al. "The mechanisms of glycemic variability accelerate diabetic central neuropathy and diabetic peripheral neuropathy in diabetic rats."

Biochemical and Biophysical Research Communications 510.1 (2019): 35–41, https://www.sciencedirect.com/science/article/abs/pii/S0006291X18328663.

Gut health

Kawano, Yoshinaga, et al. "Microbiota imbalance induced by dietary sugar disrupts immune-mediated protection from metabolic syndrome." *Cell* 185.19 (2022): 3501–3519, https://www.sciencedirect.com/science/article/abs/pii/S0092867422009928?dgcid=author.

Mineshita, Yui, et al. "Relationship between fasting and postprandial glucose levels and the gut microbiota." *Metabolites* 12.7 (2022): 669, https://www.ncbi.nlm.nih.gov/pmc/articles/PMC9319618/.

Satokari, Reetta. "High intake of sugar and the balance between pro- and anti-inflammatory gut bacteria." *Nutrients* 12.5 (2020): 1348, https://www.ncbi.nlm.nih.gov/pmc/articles/PMC7284805/.

Fertility, PCOS, hormonal issues, menopause

Bermingham, Kate M., et al. "Menopause is associated with postprandial metabolism, metabolic health, and lifestyle: The ZOE PREDICT study." *EBioMedicine* 85 (2022): 104303, https://pubmed.ncbi.nlm.nih.gov/36270905/.

Vitti, Alisa. *In the FLO: Unlock Your Hormonal Advantage and Revolutionize Your Life.* New York: HarperCollins, 2020.

Cancer

Ling, Suping, et al. "Glycosylated haemoglobin and prognosis in 10,536 people with cancer and pre-existing diabetes: A meta-analysis with dose-response analysis." *BMC Cancer* 22.1 (2022): 1–12, https://pubmed.ncbi.nlm.nih.gov/36203139/.

Alzheimer's and dementia

Abbasi, Fahim, et al. "Insulin resistance and accelerated cognitive aging." *Psychoneuroendocrinology* 147 (2023): 105944, https://pubmed.ncbi.nlm.nih.gov/36272362/.

Zhang, Xiaoling, et al. "Midlife lipid and glucose levels are associated with Alzheimer's disease." *Alzheimer's & Dementia* (2022), https://pubmed.ncbi.nlm.nih.gov/35319157/.

Jessie's disclaimer

In this book, I make existing scientific discoveries accessible to everyone. I translate them into practical tips. I am a scientist, not a doctor, so remember that none of this is medical advice. If you have a medical condition or take medication, speak to your doctor before using the hacks in this book.

Publisher's disclaimer

The material in this book is for informational purposes only. As each individual situation is unique, you should use proper discretion, in consultation with a health care practitioner, before undertaking the diet, exercise, and techniques described in this book.

The author and publisher expressly disclaim responsibility for any adverse effects that may result from the use or application of the information contained in this book.

SIMON
ELEMENT

An Imprint of Simon & Schuster, Inc.
1230 Avenue of the Americas
New York, NY 10020

Copyright © 2023 by Jessie Inchauspé

All rights reserved, including the right to reproduce this book or portions thereof in any form whatsoever. For information, address Simon Element Subsidiary Rights Department, 1230 Avenue of the Americas, New York, NY 10020.

First Simon Element hardcover edition May 2023

SIMON ELEMENT is a trademark of Simon & Schuster, Inc.

For information about special discounts for bulk purchases, please contact Simon & Schuster Special Sales at 1-866-506-1949 or business@simonandschuster.com.

The Simon & Schuster Speakers Bureau can bring authors to your live event.
For more information or to book an event, contact the Simon & Schuster Speakers Bureau at 1-866-248-3049 or visit our website at www.simonspeakers.com.

Interior design and art direction: Smith & Gilmour; recipe writer: Kathryn Bruton; recipe editor: Judy Barratt; portrait photography on pages 4, 13, 25, 103, 216, 225, 269, 270, 288: Osvaldo Ponto; food stylist: Annie Rigg; props stylist: Hannah Wilkinson

Manufactured in the United States of America

10 9 8 7 6 5 4 3 2 1

Library of Congress Control Number: 2023932926

ISBN 978-1-6680-2452-2
ISBN 978-1-6680-2453-9 (ebook)

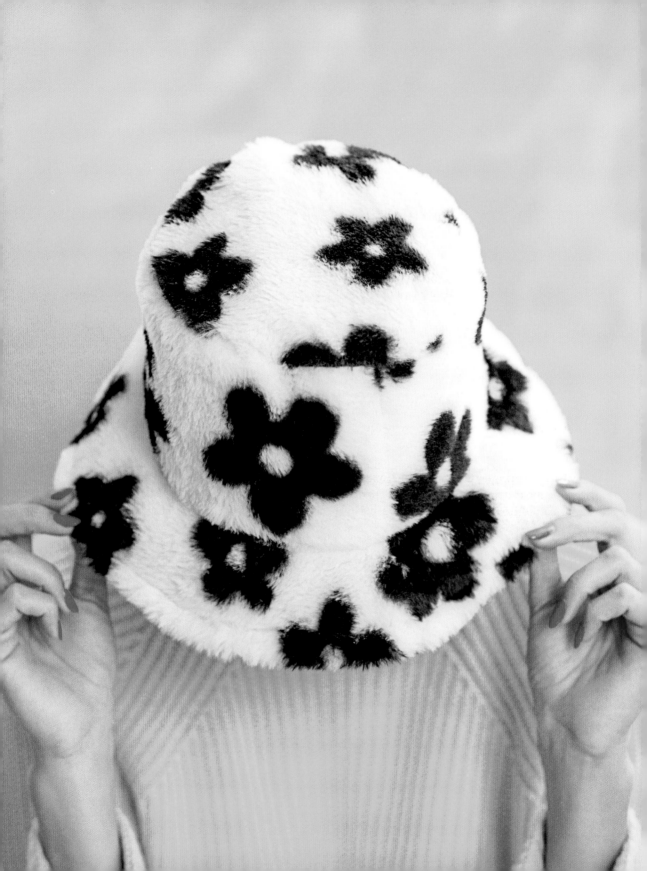

THE DREAM TEAM

The incredible people who got this book into your hands:

Kathryn Bruton, recipe fairy, who so perfectly captured the essence of *Glucose Goddess* and understood my abstract briefs, such as "This recipe is a banana in a microwave."

Alex and Emma Smith, creatives extraordinaire, who brought this book to life and lent their talent and priceless experience to this movement. It was so fun to create the world of the Glucose Goddess Method with you.

Annie Rigg and Hattie Baker, food stylists, and Hannah Wilkinson, prop stylist, who made the recipes approachable, friendly, and irresistible. Our readers feel empowered and excited to embark on this journey thanks to you.

Judy Barratt and Janey Kaspari, writers, who wrapped the text in a gorgeous bow. Thank you for making sure the message was crystal clear and the stories were delightful.

Eloisa Faltoni, Lara Hemeryck, and Justin Espedido, the backbone of the Glucose Goddess community. We wouldn't be here without you.

Aurea Carpenter and Rebecca Nicolson, my British fairy godmothers: Thank you for starting your New River adventure with me and for your kindness and support. May we always work on "the next book" together.

Leah Miller and Richard Rhorer, and everyone at Simon Elements—my American angels—who understood the power and potential of this work. Thank you for welcoming me and for taking *The Glucose Goddess Method* into your capable hands.

Sophie Rouanet and Sophie Charnavel, and everyone at Robert Laffont, my French family: Working with you has been—quite literally—like coming home. Thank you from the bottom of my heart.

Justine and Louise de Montalembert, Constance Govare and Laetitia Brun, and Eugénie Derez, the visionaries: There was a *before you,* and an *after you.* You ushered *GlucoseGoddess* into a new era. You gave her the wings that she deserved but that only you could find.

Osvaldo Ponton, my amazing photographer: Just the thought of working with you has me sigh a sigh of relief. Thank you for saying yes to my projects and for being so damn good.

My publishers, sales, and distribution teams across the globe, you are the reason this science is reaching the millions of people it is reaching. I'm honored to work with you.

Susanna Lea, my fierce and fabulous agent: I don't even know where to start to thank you. There would be no page to write thank-yous on if it weren't for you. You took me on the journey of a lifetime. Thank you for offering me this incredible opportunity to grow and reveal myself to the world. It's a gift like no other.

Everyone at SLA, working with you is a dream come true. Thank you.

And finally, Dario, the man who saw it all from the inside: I am the happiest woman in the world to be sharing my life with you. Thank you for making me pasta when I'm crying over my book covers. I love you.

INDEX

ABOUT THE AUTHOR

Jessie Inchauspé is a French biochemist and author. She is on a mission to translate cutting-edge science into easy tips to help people improve their physical and mental health. In her first book, *Glucose Revolution*, a number one international bestseller translated into 40 languages, she shared her startling discovery about the essential role of blood sugar in every aspect of our lives, and the surprising hacks to optimize it. Jessie is the founder of the wildly popular Instagram account @GlucoseGoddess, where she teaches more than one million people about transformative food habits. She holds a BSc in mathematics from King's College, London, and an MSc in biochemistry from Georgetown University.

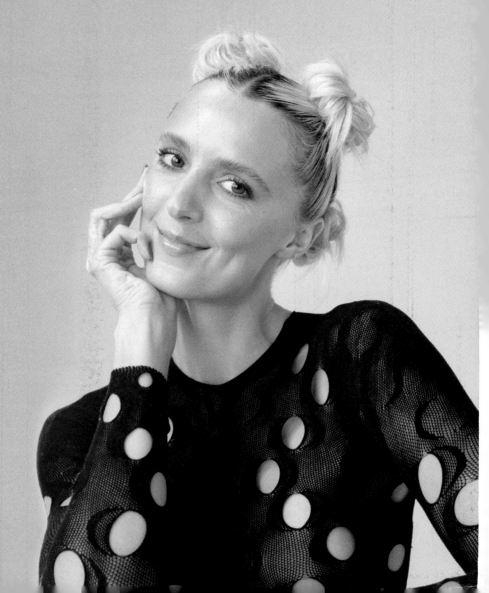